Understanding your
Bowels

George F. Longstreth M.D.
Ken W. Heaton M.D.

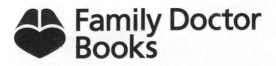

Family Doctor Books

IMPORTANT
This book is intended not as a substitute for personal
medical advice but as a supplement to that advice for
the patient who wishes to understand more about his
or her condition.

Before taking any form of treatment
YOU SHOULD ALWAYS CONSULT YOUR MEDICAL
PRACTITIONER.

In particular (without limit) you should note that advances
in medical science occur rapidly and some information
about medication and treatment contained in this booklet
may very soon be out of date.

ISBN-10: 1-4285-0012-X
ISBN-13: 978-1-4285-0012-9

Contents

About the authors

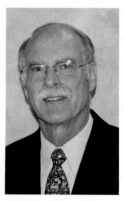

Dr. George F. Longstreth is Chief of Gastroenterology with the Kaiser Permanente Medical Care Plan in San Diego, California and Clinical Professor of Medicine at the University of California San Diego School of Medicine. He has published about 100 scientific papers, chaired the Functional Bowel Committee of the Rome III International Working Teams, and is Past President of the Functional Brain-Gut Research Group.

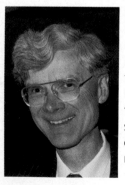

Dr. Ken Heaton was until recently Reader in Medicine at the University of Bristol, United Kingdom and Honorary Consultant Physician to the United Bristol Hospitals Trust. His research interests are in bowel function and nutrition. He has served on many national committees and has published nearly 300 scientific papers.

Introduction

Attitudes about your bowels

From childhood, many of us are conditioned to think of stools as dirty and disgusting. Children learn early to use substitute words for "bowel movements" such as "BM" or "number 2," and some people are reluctant to discuss bowel function after they grow up. There are

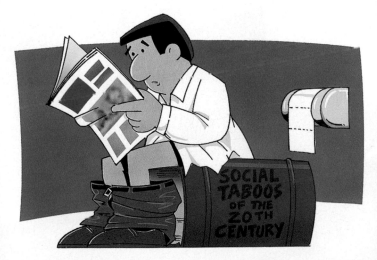

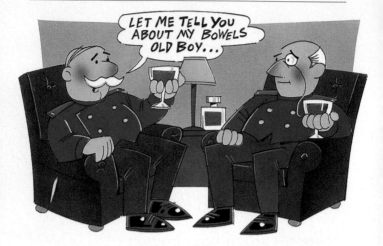

people who avoid looking at their own stools. Bowel movements occur in private, and who has not been embarrassed by passing gas in the company of others?

On the other hand, some people are becoming less inhibited about these matters. For example, a 43-year-

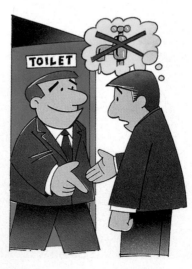

old manicurist recently told a client, "My friends used to just talk about sex and men. Now we talk about our poop." Such discussions are not limited to the elderly. Less secrecy can be a good thing, but it won't help if people don't understand what they are talking about.

Deficient knowledge is widespread concerning the bowels. The colon and rectum are mysterious. Most people know more about the heart. Yet nearly everyone has occasional diarrhea or hemorrhoids, and many people have chronic bowel symptoms that make them concerned they may have a serious condition. Depending on your knowledge, you could repeatedly seek medical care for non-threatening symptoms or delay proper evaluation of a problem that is serious. This booklet explains how the bowels work and why they give you trouble. It will help prevent problems and let you know what to do if problems occur.

KEY POINTS

■ Biased attitudes about the bowels date from early childhood.

■ Bowel disorders are extremely common, yet people vary as to their willingness to discuss bowel matters and their knowledge of them

■ Increased knowledge can help you prevent and cope with bowel problems

A brief guide to the bowels

Some words and phrases

The word "bowels" is one of those vague words that can mean different things to different people. Doctors use it to describe both the large and small intestines. Often, as in this book, the term is limited to the large

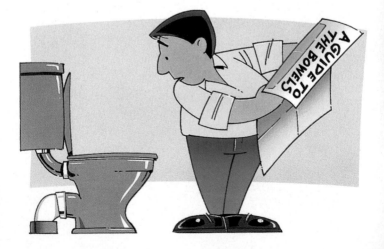

intestine or colon and rectum, which is the last part of the gastrointestinal tract. More medical terms are explained in the Glossary on pages 113–117.

Bowel movements

When people speak of "moving the bowels" or "having a bowel movement," they are trying to speak politely of the activity which is correctly called defecation. Another less technical way of saying this is "passing stool." Stools and feces mean the same thing to doctors. These words are rarely used in polite conversation; most people use roundabout expressions instead, such as "using the bathroom," which is imprecise as it applies to both urination and defecation.

Passing gas

The correct term for gas passed from the rectum is "flatus." Many people refer to it as "gas," but this is imprecise because "gas" can also mean upper

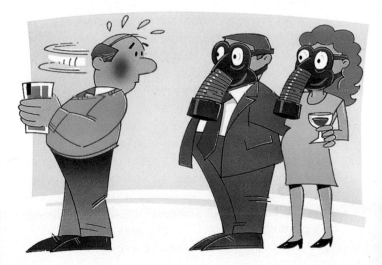

abdominal discomfort, abdominal distension, gurgling noise, heartburn, or belching (burping). "Fart" has the advantage of meaning only one thing, but many people regard this as vulgar. Probably the nearest we have to an expression that is both unambiguous and reasonably polite is "passing gas."

The large intestine

The large intestine consists of the colon, rectum, and anal canal (see illustration on page 7). The colon begins just above the right groin where it is known as the cecum; the appendix extends off it and can become seriously inflamed (the condition known as appendicitis). It continues as the ascending colon, which climbs to just below the ribs on the right and then swings across to the opposite side as the transverse colon. With a second sharp bend it turns downward as the descending colon, and finally makes a curious loop known as the sigmoid (named after the squiggly Greek letter sigma or Σ) before becoming the last part, the rectum.

The word "rectum" comes from the Latin word for "straight," which is odd because actually it bends sharply backward just before it joins the anal canal. It straightens out, however, during bowel movements, when it functions simply as a tube conducting stools from the sigmoid colon to the toilet.

Strictly speaking, it is the anal canal that does the last part of this job, but the canal is only an inch or so long and is really just a device for keeping stools and gas inside until we decide to let them out. The anal canal, like the throat, has muscles like those in our arms and legs, which we can voluntarily control. The gastrointestinal tract is mainly controlled by its own nervous system (the enteric nervous system), which is affected by connections to the main (central) nervous system and by various hormones that act through the bloodstream.

The anal muscle fibers are arranged as a two-part closing system. First, there is a sling of fibers around the upper end of the tube. When this muscle contracts it exerts a forward pull and so maintains the sharp angle where the rectum joins the anus; at the same time, it presses the front and back of the canal against each

The parts of the bowels

Food travels from the stomach, through the small intestine to the large intestine. It travels up the ascending colon where it is fermented, then across the transverse colon where water and salt are removed. It is stored in the descending colon and sigmoid colon, and passes to the rectum, along the anal canal and out of the anus when you have a bowel movement.

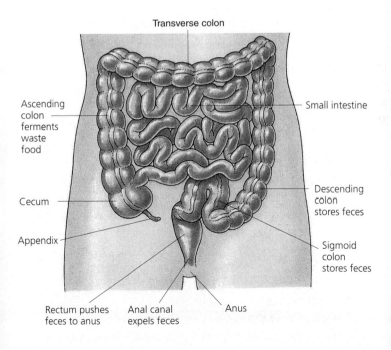

Transverse colon

Ascending colon ferments waste food

Small intestine

Cecum

Descending colon stores feces

Appendix

Sigmoid colon stores feces

Rectum pushes feces to anus

Anal canal expels feces

Anus

other. Second, there is a ring of fibers whose contraction narrows the opening in the tubular bowel.

Both sets of fibers are contracting gently all the time without any conscious effort on our part (just like many other muscles in the body). We have to relax these muscles in order to pass a stool or gas. Some people find this difficult (see page 57).

The lining of the bowel

Digestion, the breaking down of food into protein, fat, carbohydrate, vitamins, and other nutrients that can be absorbed, occurs in the stomach and small intestine. The large intestine converts dietary waste to solid stools that can be eliminated conveniently. It does this by absorbing water and salts (especially sodium) through its lining (mucosa) between the muscular wall and the interior of the bowel (lumen). The skin on the outside joins this lining inside the anus. Large numbers of benefical bacteria are also added in the colon to increase stool bulk.

This fragile lining has the difficult task of acting as a barrier to dangerous bacteria and viruses while, at the same time, letting through into the bloodstream beneficial substances such as water and salts to prevent us from becoming dehydrated.

It is a balancing act. If the mucosa absorbs too much water, the stools become hard and difficult to pass; if it absorbs too little, they are liquid and copious and the anal muscles have difficulty keeping them in. At one extreme there is constipation, at the other, diarrhea and incontinence (loss of control of bowel movements).

Movements

The muscles of the bowel seldom rest—every few seconds they contract briefly in short sections of bowel.

These contractions make the bowel narrower and drive its contents forward and backward into neighboring sections which are relaxed. Most of these movements simply shuttle the contents back and forth, presumably to increase their exposure to the mucosa and ensure the maximum absorption of important water and salts.

Now and again, a strong wave of contraction passes through the entire colon, pushing its contents toward the rectum. This is known as *peristalsis* or mass movement, and it occurs mostly after meals and in the morning after awakening , This explains why many people feel the need to have a bowel movement after breakfast or even sooner after getting out of bed. A cup of tea or coffee can also have this effect.

Sensations

The fortunate among us experience sensations from our bowel only when we need to pass stools or gas. In both cases, the sensations are signals from the rectum,

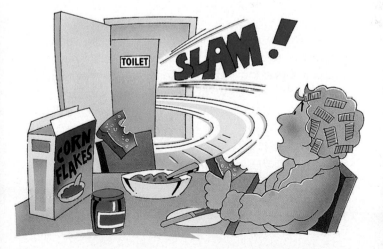

How the bowel muscles work

When the muscles in the bowel wall contract, they move the contents along. When short sections contract and then relax, the contents move back and forth. If the contractions follow each other in a wave along the length of the bowel, the contents are moved towards the rectum. The difference is not in the strength of the contraction but in whether it keeps moving in the same direction, towards the rectum.

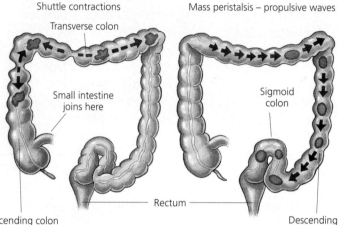

Shuttle contractions

Mass peristalsis – propulsive waves

Transverse colon

Small intestine joins here

Sigmoid colon

Rectum

Ascending colon

Descending colon

indicating that it is receiving material from the sigmoid colon. The amazing thing is that we can tell from the signal whether the material is solid, liquid, or gaseous, and we can pass gas without evacuating stool. The distinction is probably made by miniature sensors at the top end of the anal canal.

Many people also feel wriggling movements in their abdomen when gas is moved from one part of the colon to another. At the same time, a gurgling sound may be heard. Other people feel a wave of discomfort, which may even be painful, when the need to have a bowel movement is strong, for example, if the stool is

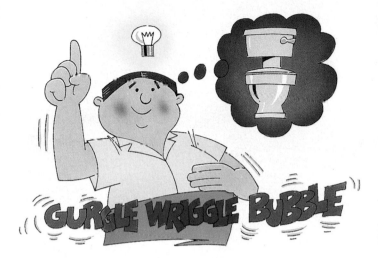

looser than usual. All these sensations are perfectly normal, up to a point.

Discomfort and pain from the colon are extremely common in otherwise healthy people (see Irritable bowel syndrome, page 82). Usually this implies that the bowel is contracting strongly or that the bowel has become more sensitive for some reason.

Bacteria: friends and foes

A unique feature of the large intestine is that it is host to a huge number of bacteria. In fact, about 60% of the solid portion of stool consists of bacteria, comprising about 500 different species. The bacteria set up residence in early infancy and, although they vary from one person to another, they remain mostly unchanged throughout life unless disturbed by antibiotics, diarrhea, or dietary change. Not only are most of them harmless, they even provide important

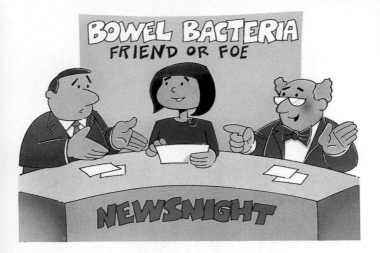

benefits. Normal bacteria ferment non-digestible dietary residue in the right side of the colon, producing certain acids that provide the energy the large intestine needs to do its work. This is where much of the gas comes from that is passed as flatus. Bacteria also help control the growth of the mucosa and are integral to the development of an immune system that protects us throughout life, in contrast to bacteria-free laboratory animals whose defective immune system predisposes them to infectious diseases. Finally, they protect us from the ill effects of the periodic ingestion of harmful bacteria.

So, by all means, respect your bowel bacteria but do not live in fear of them. Most of them are good for us. Probiotics are bacteria with special health benefits. For example, *Lactobacilli* in yogurt enable people with intolerance to milk sugar (lactose) to consume this milk product comfortably.

Bowel bacteria can cause illness

If colonic bacteria have a bad reputation, it is not because of the gas they produce, but for one of the following reasons:

- When, through injury or disease, the bacteria get into other parts of the body, they can produce infections such as bladder inflammation (known as cystitis).

- When poor hygiene allows one person's colonic bacteria to get into another person's food or drink this can cause gastroenteritis (inflammation with diarrhea). A common example is travelers' diarrhea.

- Antibiotics sometimes kill the friendly bacteria and allow harmful bacteria to proliferate, especially *Clostridium difficile*, which causes severe diarrhea from inflammation of the large bowel (a condition known as colitis).

Bowel movements—what is normal?

The large bowel and its products have never been popular subjects for research so, not surprisingly, scientific data on them are limited. However, we know the following facts and figures about normal adults.

Many people claim to pass stools once a day but, when they are asked to record all their bowel movements, it turns out that a regular daily bowel habit is present in fewer than 50% of people. About 96% of people have between three movements a day and three movements a week. However, some people's bowel frequency is within this normal range, but they have bothersome urgency or difficulty passing stool. Therefore, simple frequency is not the only factor of importance. The average passage time of undigested food residues through the human gut is about 50 hours in men and 57 hours in women, but ranges from well under 20 to over 100 hours. It also changes from one day to the next. Most of this time (80 to 90%) is spent in the colon. The goal is not to have a bowel movement every day but to pass stools without distress. Even a once-daily habit is no guarantee that all is well. It is possible to go once a day but with such slow passage that every evacuation is four or five days late and stools are hard and painful to pass. A better guide to passage time than frequency of bowel movements is the appearance of the stool.

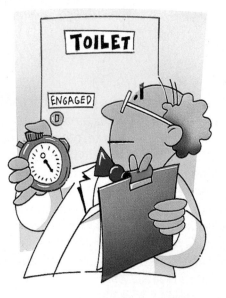

Progress of food through the body

After swallowing, food is moved by muscular contractions through the digestive system. The time spent in each part depends on the stage of digestion. It also varies with food type and quantity, and from day to day. The usual total time can vary from 15 hours to 5 days.

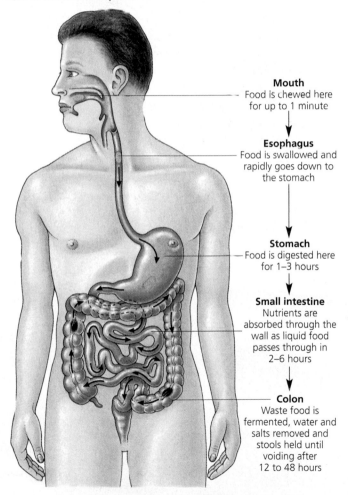

Mouth
Food is chewed here for up to 1 minute

Esophagus
Food is swallowed and rapidly goes down to the stomach

Stomach
Food is digested here for 1–3 hours

Small intestine
Nutrients are absorbed through the wall as liquid food passes through in 2–6 hours

Colon
Waste food is fermented, water and salts removed and stools held until voiding after 12 to 48 hours

Types of stool

Medical specialists classified stool into seven types, on what is called the Bristol Stool Form Scale (see below), according to their appearance as seen in the toilet. Type 1 has spent the most time in the colon and type 7 the least time.

Stools at the lumpy end of the scale are hard to pass and often require a lot of straining. Stools at the loose or liquid end of the range can be too easy to pass—the need to pass them is urgent and accidents can happen. The ideal stools are in the middle of the range, especially type 4, as they are most likely to glide out easily. Also, they are least likely to leave you with an annoying feeling that something is left behind.

Stool color

Stools are usually some shade of brown, but green and yellow colors may sometimes appear, depending on the

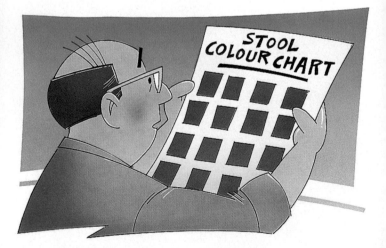

The Bristol Stool Form Scale

This chart lists the range of stool types most commonly passed.

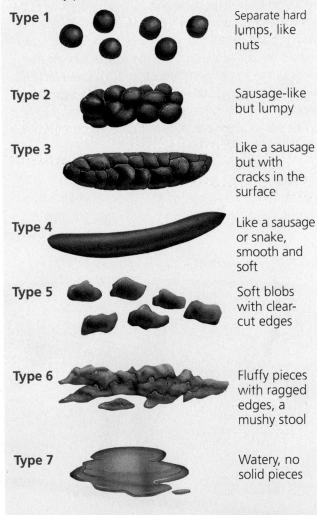

Type 1 — Separate hard lumps, like nuts

Type 2 — Sausage-like but lumpy

Type 3 — Like a sausage but with cracks in the surface

Type 4 — Like a sausage or snake, smooth and soft

Type 5 — Soft blobs with clear-cut edges

Type 6 — Fluffy pieces with ragged edges, a mushy stool

Type 7 — Watery, no solid pieces

diet and other factors. Bismuth (as in Pepto-Bismol) and iron supplements turn them black. Aside from beet ingestion that can color stools red and bits of tomato skin, blood is what usually makes stools red. This can be a sign of serious disease requiring medical care, but it is often attributable to harmless bleeding from hemorrhoids. Black stools resembling tar are typically caused by loss of blood from the stomach or nearby areas in the upper gastrointestinal tract that blackens on its way through the bowel. This usually signifies serious bleeding, often from an ulcer, is often accompanied by weakness, and calls for prompt medical attention.

Flatus

The average person passes gas 12 times in 24 hours. This fact was established in young men, and the

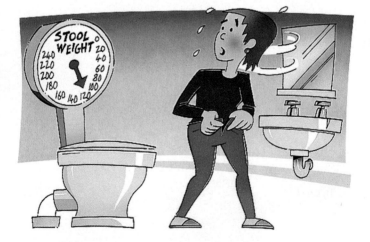

situation may be different in older people and in women. There is a great deal of person-to-person variation that partly depends on the fermentation activity of bacteria on the non-digestible dietary waste in the bowel .

The mysteries remaining

The lack of basic scientific data in this field of human experience is extraordinary. For example, we do not know how long people spend over the act of defecation. It is widely taught that straining (holding the breath and pushing) is a normal and necessary part of defecation. However, recent research has shown that straining is a minority practice and, what's more, depends on the type, size, and consistency of the stool.

The ideal bowel movement

The features listed here are all likely to accompany the passing of a Type 4 stool (see the Bristol Stool Form Scale on page 17).

- The feeling that you need to "go" is definite but not irresistible
- Once you sit down on the toilet there is no delay
- No conscious effort or straining is needed
- The stool glides out smoothly and comfortably
- Afterwards there is only a pleasant feeling of relief

KEY POINTS

- The large intestine comprises the colon, the rectum, and the anal canal. The only part we consciously control is the anal canal

- The lining of the large intestine absorbs water and salts and repels bacteria and viruses

- To aid absorption, the intestines constantly move the contents back and forth as well as downward

- Intestinal bacteria nourish the colon and are a valuable defense against disease, even though they also produce gas

- How often we have bowel movements varies greatly; most of us do not have a precise 24-hour cycle

- Many aspects of the bowels are still a mystery

Mind and bowel— a network of interactions

Are the mind and bowel connected?

The seventeenth-century French philosopher Decartes claimed that the mind and body are separate, a dictum that influenced physicians for over 300 years, to the disadvantage of people with bowel problems. If doctors

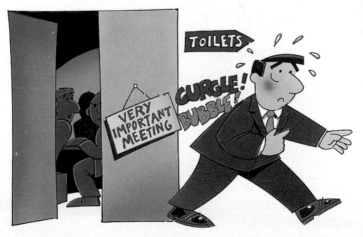

did not find an anatomical or metabolic cause for a person's symptoms, they tended to deny that the person was ill or the person was stigmatized as having purely psychological problems. Only recently have medical practitioners realized that both physical and mental factors are involved in all illnesses. Many people have serious trouble from functional bowel disorders, which lack a conventional disease cause, especially the irritable bowel syndrome (see page 82).

The bowel and brain are connected by a complex nervous system, and there are additional hormonal influences from the brain that affect the gastrointestinal tract through the bloodstream. The mind affects the bowel and the bowel affects the mind in many ways. There would probably be no need for this book if this were not true. Some effects are obvious, some are subtle. Let us look at them in turn, starting with the neglected but important matter of how the bowel affects the mind.

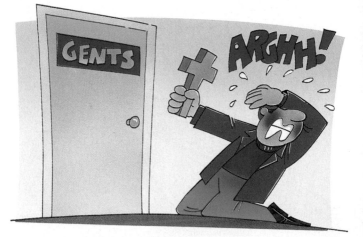

Attitudes to the bowel

All the internal organs of the body are mysterious to
non-medical people but this does not stop people from
having feelings about them. Take the heart and the
brain. Everyone, quite rightly, thinks the heart and brain
are marvelous inventions of nature; our feelings about
them are positive, even warm. Take the uterus (the
womb). Women treasure the uterus as the place in
which human life begins.

Towards other organs, such as the liver and kidneys,
we have no special emotions, except perhaps gratitude
that they quietly do their jobs. The bladder can be a
source of discomfort but one that is quickly relieved
and forgotten.

Only the gastrointestinal tract evokes consistently
negative emotions.

Embarrassment

Intestines are forever drawing attention to themselves in
ways that embarrass or harass us. They gurgle loudly in
public places. They discharge a smelly gas when we are
near others. They demand attention unpredictably and in
inconvenient places. Who has not been forced to creep
away from a social or professional occasion because of
an irresistible need to have a bowel movement?

Fear of disease

And all this is when the bowel is healthy and working
normally. How much worse these things are when the
bowel is diseased or malfunctioning! And everyone
knows that the bowel is a place where serious diseases
happen. Most people have heard about bowel cancer
and many people have heard of someone who has died
of it. Indeed about 1 out of 20 Americans will get

cancer of the colon or rectum. So the seeds of fear are sown and, in many people's minds, this fear grows every time their bowels misbehave or they see a streak of blood on the toilet tissue. Screening tests for colorectal cancer are being performed more frequently, and such negative testing can go a long way to reduce anxiety.

Shame

Negative feelings of embarrassment, shame, and fear are embedded in people's attitudes about stools and defecation, that are often expressed only in negative language. One of the worst insults imaginable is to call someone "a shit." The most degrading infirmity of the human body is being unable to control one's own bowel movements.

Ignorance and denial

Ignorance leads to fear and denial. Many people are ignorant of what their stools look like; they never look

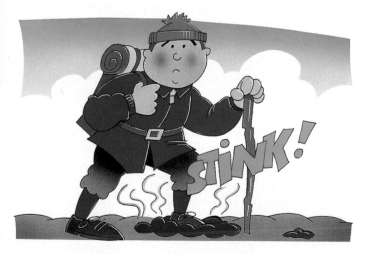

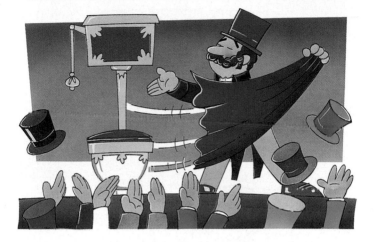

at them. This is odd because we all know what horse manure, dog feces, and bird droppings look like.

Ignorance about the act of defecation is equally profound. This normal, natural function is, simply, never discussed. Novels describe every human activity in intimate detail except for one. In books, it seems no one ever defecates. The English language—so rich in every other way—is totally deficient here. The very word "defecation" is absent from *Roget's Thesaurus of English Words and Phrases.*

The only words most people know are the crude words "crap" and "shit," or such childish euphemisms as "number two." In the English-speaking world there is a conspiracy of denial.

To summarize, in our culture, people's attitudes to the intestines and their products are expressed as disgust, embarrassment, shame, fear, and denial. These negative attitudes color the way we react to bowel problems.

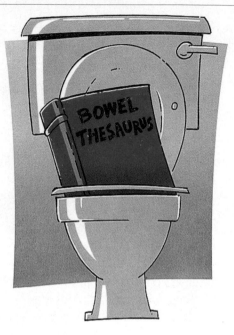

How the mind affects the bowel

All human beings experience strong emotions that can affect every function of the body. A severe shock can make a person faint; it can make their heart race. Anger can turn people's faces red or white and make them shake uncontrollably. Anxiety makes people feel hot while fear makes them break into a cold sweat. Knees buckle, heads spin, eyes gush fluid, mouths go dry, throats go tight, voices go hoarse—all these things happen as a result of emotion.

The effects of emotion on the body are mostly on organs that are outside our conscious control. Our intestines certainly belong in this category. Experiments performed on volunteers using endoscopes, balloons, and pressure-recording devices have proved that fear can paralyze the lower bowel and anger can work it up into a frenzy of activity. Everyday experience bears this out. The student waiting to go into an exam, the applicant before an interview, the athlete before a game, the soldier before a battle—all are likely to have a violent urge to pass a loose stool.

Stress and pent-up emotions such as fear, anger, and resentment can have widely differing effects—in some people less frequent bowel movements and lumpier stools, in others more frequent movements and looser stools. Age and sex affect this reaction, as about 50% of younger (less than 45 years of age) women report a stress effect on bowel pattern compared with about 30% of younger men, and both

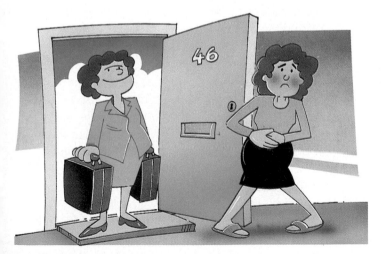

women and men report less of this stress effect as they grow older—an unrecognized benefit of aging for some people! Many people under stress develop the discomfort and abnormal stools of the irritable bowel syndrome. They then become anxious about their insides and this causes further disturbances of bowel function.

What happens in all these examples is that emotional reactions are internalized. Elemental feelings are expressed inwardly rather than outwardly. Instead of fists being clenched or faces turning red, the intestine clenches itself and rushes stool through. Instead of insults or missiles being thrown, the contents of the intestine are speeded onward. We cannot eliminate our gut reactions, but we can modify them and cope with their effects.

Bowels and the stresses of modern life

Civilization saves us from the cruder stresses of animal life or of primitive man—at least in times of peace. However, modern life creates new stresses that are more subtle and, perhaps, more difficult to cope with. For one thing, society demands that we hide our feelings—except at funerals and sports events! We say that we are controlling ourselves but all we are doing is hiding our feelings. Feelings cannot be wished away and, if we hide them, they will still affect us in some way.

Having to control our reactions is stressful, yet failure to do so can incur disapproval or disgrace. We all need to learn coping tactics but few of us are taught them.

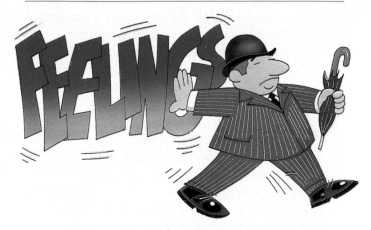

Talking with other people about our feelings is often helpful, but this is not always easy. There may be nobody available with whom we want to discuss them. Many people, especially men, are reluctant to talk about their feelings because they have learned to deny their existence. They have buried their feelings so deeply that they have lost touch with them. Not expressing feelings makes it more likely that the internal organs of the body will show the effects of stress.

The vicious cycle of symptoms

Let us look now at what can happen when, for one reason or another, someone's intestinal function is disturbed. There are many reasons why this could happen besides a stressful event, as described on page 26.

Considering the negative reaction that bowels and stools induce in many of us, it is easy to see how fear and anxiety induced by symptoms affect the workings of the intestine and make those symptoms worse. Continuation of the symptoms reinforces the negative emotions, especially the fear that there is something seriously wrong, and the continuing negative emotions reinforce the symptoms.

And so it goes, especially if the sufferer has a friend or relative who had cancer of the bowel or other serious disease that appeared to cause similar symptoms—but you don't know if other features of their illness made it different from yours in important ways. A vicious cycle like this can be broken if the sufferer is quickly seen by a knowledgeable doctor or other healthcare professional. The origin and meaning of the symptoms can be explained and the individual reassured that they have a common, everyday occurrence that often improves, at least if it is not worried about.

A missed opportunity

Unfortunately, this often does not happen, for several reasons. The sufferer may be too shy or too busy to seek help. Or he or she might fail to explain the symptoms accurately. Sometimes the doctor doesn't listen closely enough or is brusque and unsympathetic, and the opportunity for reassurance is lost.

This is particularly bad because the sufferer realizes that his or her sufferings have been misunderstood and wonders "What do I do now? Why didn't he listen to me? Was it my fault? Dare I ask to see the doctor again?" This extra layer of emotions perpetuates and strengthens the vicious cycle.

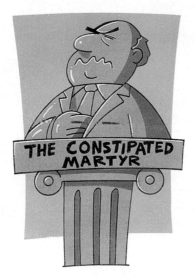

Physical pain instead of mental anguish

There are more subtle reasons why symptoms can
persist. Physical pain can be easier to bear than
psychological pain. If the pain started as a response to
life's stresses, it may be a substitute for anger or anxiety
and be easier to bear than the original raw emotion. If
the underlying stress has not been addressed, the
sufferer could unconsciously choose to have pain rather
than to feel the raw emotion.

In modern life, there are many intractable conflicts—
between the older and younger generations, between
staff and bosses, between family and working longer
hours, and so on. Conflicts create tension and long-
standing tension can turn into chronic anxiety or
depression.

It may be socially less acceptable to complain of

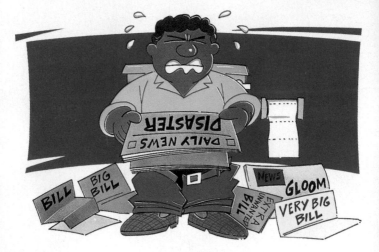

anxiety or depression or other forms of mental pain than to complain of physical pain and other bodily symptoms. People with physical problems may be perceived as victims of forces outside themselves and deserving of sympathy, whereas people with mental complaints may be perceived as weak and just needing to "get a grip."

No wonder abdominal pain and other stress-related bowel symptoms are so common. Surveys show that many people with these problems have difficulty coping with life.

How does mental distress cause intestinal symptoms?

The body's computer systems for receiving signals from the intestines, analyzing them, and telling the intestine what to do are immensely complex and far from fully understood. The brain, where all sensations are registered, including those from the intestine, controls events in the gastrointestinal tract indirectly and unconsciously. It operates through another nervous system which is embedded in the intestine, the enteric nervous system (ENS). The ENS needs no help from above in controlling the intestine; in fact, it functions most smoothly if left to its own devices. Mental states affect the intestine by altering the controls in the ENS.

Signals or messages coming down from the brain make the ENS more sensitive, reacting to weak stimuli as if they were strong ones. Current research suggests that the nerve endings or receptors in the intestinal wall are "up-regulated" (the current jargon for "placed on red alert"), but there may also be changes in the "junction boxes." These appear to allow weaker than normal signals through, and the signals may even be amplified so that they get all the way up the spinal cord to the brain.

There are similar junction boxes in the spinal cord where incoming signals from the intestine can get amplified when the wrong messages or too many

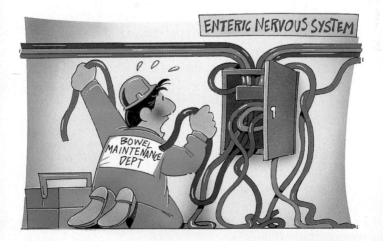

ENTERIC NERVOUS SYSTEM

BOWEL MAINTENANCE DEPT

The nervous control of bowel movements

The digestive system has its own nervous system, called the
enteric nervous system or ENS. We cannot affect our bowels
consciously but emotions can cause the system to misbehave and
the effects can be long-lasting.

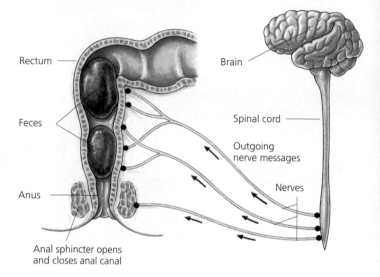

Rectum

Feces

Anus

Anal sphincter opens
and closes anal canal

Brain

Spinal cord

Outgoing
nerve messages

Nerves

messages come down from the brain. In the higher
centers of the brain, lines can get crossed so that signals
from the intestine get mixed up with emotional feelings.

The exact mechanisms are not fully worked out, but
advanced tests of brain function are starting to reveal
them. We know that, after a time, the settings of
junction boxes in the nervous system can become fixed
so that, long after the original intestinal upset or
mental problem has disappeared, the mechanisms still
exist for producing abnormal sensations from the
intestine. It is as if a pain or other symptom becomes
imprinted on the nervous system. In this way the pain
becomes chronic and intractable.

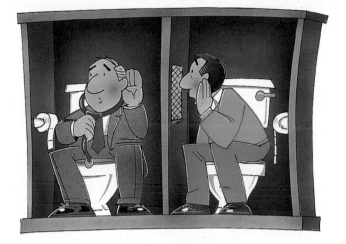

What can be done?

People can avoid vicious cycles and intractable symptoms by keeping calm and not jumping to pessimistic conclusions every time they have a pain in the abdomen, a hard stool, or a series of loose stools. Remember that these things happen all the time to countless people, that they usually have no sinister significance, and that they usually disappear on their own. Look at the list of common causes of short-lived intestinal malfunction (see page 87) and ask yourself if one of them seems to apply. If so, expect things to get better.

If they don't or, for any other reason, you decide to see your doctor, make sure that he or she really understands what you are saying is wrong with you. Make sure, too, that you understand the doctor's explanation about the nature of your problem. Don't be shy about your symptoms and don't be afraid to ask questions. If you can't communicate well with your doctor, consider visiting a different one. You need a therapeutic relationship with your physician. A trouble shared is a trouble halved.

KEY POINTS

- Thinking about our bowels encourages negative feelings—embarrassment, shame, and fear. These lead to denial and ignorance

- Strong emotional reactions, especially when repressed, can play havoc with the bowels

- Beware the vicious cycle: negative attitudes increase the nervous sensitivity of the bowels, magnify the feeling of intestinal discomfort, and increase anxiety and uncertainty

- A positive approach is therapeutic in itself. A therapeutic relationship with your physician is paramount

What else affects the bowels?

Time of day

The most important time of the day, as far as the bowel is concerned, is the first hour after you get up in the morning. Getting out of bed sends a wake-up message to the muscles of the colon. The movements, which

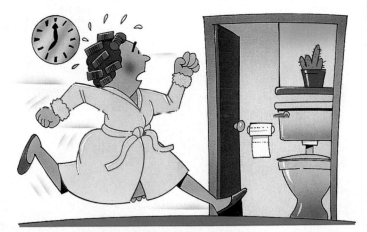

have rested overnight, resume propelling the contents of the colon toward the rectum.

In some people the drive is so powerful that the rectum fills and, within minutes of getting up, they get an urge to "go." In many people, the wake-up effect on the colon is less strong and has to be reinforced by breakfast. Eating food at any time of day first arouses the stomach, which also sends a reflex message to the colon to move more.

A morning routine is important for many people. If the urge to go before or after breakfast is strong, well and good—it is unlikely to be ignored. However, if the feeling is less powerful, so that the person is not forced to go and happens to be in a hurry or is emotionally stressed, then the urge is liable to be ignored.

Encourage a regular habit

The urge may also be ignored if it delays its appearance until you are on the way to work or have begun the

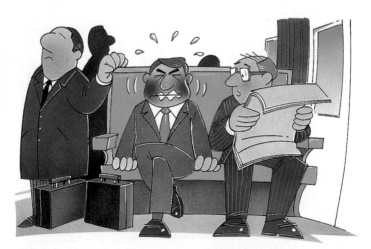

day's activities. It is all too easy to suppress the bowel urge then, and it may go away and not come back for several hours or even a whole day.

Obeying the bowel urge is the first essential for getting a regular bowel habit and a regular routine, which is also more likely if breakfast is not neglected. A bowel urge that is regularly expected and regularly acted upon is most likely to make its appearance regularly. On the other hand, any change in routine, such as traveling, can completely abolish the usual habit and retard bowel activity.

Physical exercise

Many people become constipated if they are confined to bed due to illness or injury. At the other extreme, marathon runners sometimes get diarrhea during a race. It is widely believed that being physically active

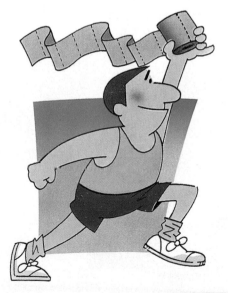

helps to prevent constipation, but the scientific evidence is meager. Nevertheless, physical activity has many other benefits and is recommended to promote general health.

Dietary fiber and starch

Of all the things we eat, fiber is especially important to the workings of the large intestine, Dietary fiber comes from the cell walls of plants mainly in the form of cellulose and related molecules (chemical substances). Starch, a related substance, comes from inside the plant cells.

We digest most of the starch in the small intestine, but dietary fiber escapes digestion, so it reaches the colon along with small amounts of undigested starch, bile, and other liquids that are added to it during passage.

This process creates about 3 pints (1½ liters) of a thick soup-like material a day that enters the large

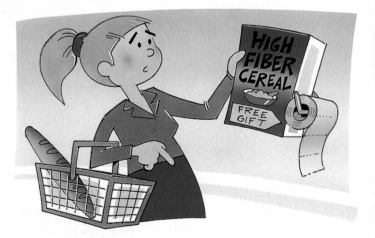

intestine. The colon converts this into a thick paste of spongy-solid material by absorbing most of the water and by the complex process of bacterial fermentation.

Fermentation

Fermentation is a chain of events whereby the large molecules in dietary fiber and starch are broken down into small, simple ones by the bacteria in the colon. The bacteria do this in order to obtain energy for their own growth and multiplication, but there are two remarkable spin-offs—gases and acids.

Gases

The gases are known to all of us because we pass gas every day. They consist of hydrogen and carbon dioxide and, in some people, methane. The bad odor comes from bacterial breakdown of protein. Although the gases can be inflammable, they are unlikely to be ignited!

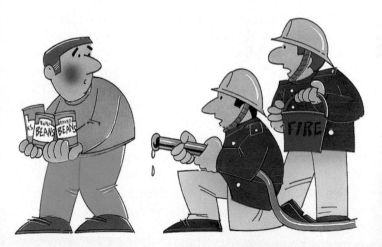

Acids

You would not normally associate the colon with vinegar but, in fact, the main acid in vinegar, acetic acid, is also the main acid in the colon. Together with two others, acetic acid is responsible for the fact that the right side of the colon where most of the fermentation takes place is so acidic that many types of bacteria cannot live there, and the growth of others is retarded. This acidity may be one of the body's defenses against harmful bacteria, such as those that cause travelers' diarrhea. One of the acids is also used as an energy source by the cells that line the colon.

Benefits of fiber

As a result of this, scientists are realizing that, to stay healthy, the colon needs to be fed with lots of fermentable material. This implies that our diet should contain lots of non-digestible fiber (except for people with unusually sensitive colons). One benefit is a plentiful supply of acids to control the population of bacteria and nourish the colon lining; the other is that stools are bulkier and softer, which makes them easier to pass.

This laxative effect of fiber has been known since antiquity but, curiously, we still do not fully understand it. Probably, several different things happen. One is that fiber acts like a sponge—it is good at holding water. Another is that it tickles the nerve endings in the bowel wall, triggering electrical circuits or reflexes that make the bowel contract. A third way is that it provides a feast for the bacteria in the bowel, which then multiply furiously and add themselves to the outgoing stool, making it bulkier. Thus, fiber is three things to the colon, all beginning with the letter S: a sponge, a stimulus, and a sacrifice.

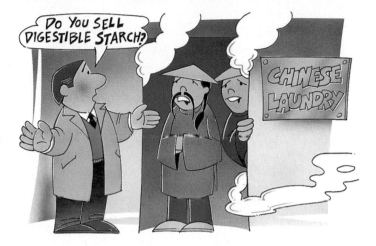

Types of fiber

The cellulose and related molecules of plant cell
walls consist mainly of huge molecules called
polysaccharides. They are formed from lots of
small sugar molecules joined end-to-end (Greek:
poly = many, saccharides = sugars). These non-starch
polysaccharides have sugar links that are hard to
split; bacteria can do it, but our digestive enzymes
cannot.

Many non-starch polysaccharides have a branching
structure that allows them to dissolve in water (soluble
fiber) and behave like gums or jellies. The pectin in
fruits, that makes Jello set, is a familiar example.

Soluble fiber is readily fermented by colon bacteria.
Insoluble fiber does not dissolve and is not fermented
well but increases the bulk of stool. It occurs in
legumes, seeds, vegetables, whole wheat, and wheat
bran. Some foods contain both types.

Sources of fiber

All foods originating from plants contain fiber provided they have not been extensively processed. In fact, the only plant-based foods that don't contain fiber are oils, sugars, and syrups. A lot of fiber is removed, however, in the refining of foods, such as the milling of white flour and white rice, and in making cornstarch and cornflakes.

The fiber-rich foods are bread, breakfast cereals, and other foods made with whole-wheat flour, and nuts, peas, beans, and lentils.

Fruits and vegetables consist mostly of water so, weight for weight, they are low in fiber. They can make an important contribution to the fiber intake if consumed daily in generous amounts, and they provide important nutrients.

The diet should include a limited intake of red meats, saturated fats, refined carbohydrates, and

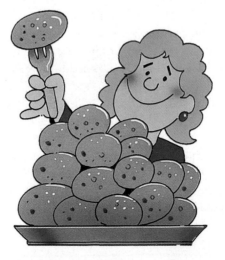

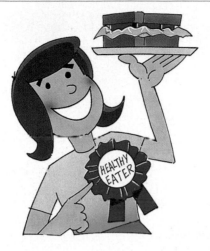

alcohol. Fiber-rich foods also supply beneficial antioxidant vitamins and folic acid, and dairy foods or other calcium sources are also needed. This type of diet reduces the possibility of getting diabetes, heart disease, colon cancer, and other diseases, as well as obesity.

Laxative foods

Tables showing the fiber content of different foods are a limited guide to their laxative effect. People vary in how foods affect them. Furthermore, foods vary in their effect, depending on how they have been handled and cooked, and even on how old or ripe they are. So, to get the right amount of fiber, it is best to depend on general principles: maintain a low intake of oils, sugars, and syrups (and animal fats), and keep up your intake of unprocessed or lightly processed plant foods.

Some people need more fiber than they can easily get from whole-wheat cereals so, to avoid constipation,

Amounts of fiber contained in some foods

Food and portion size	Dietary fiber (g)
Breads and cereals	
All Bran, ⅓ cup	8.5
Bran (100%), ½ cup	8.4
Corn Bran, ⅔ cup	5.4
Bran Chex, ⅔ cup	4.6
Oatmeal, 1 cup	2.2
Whole-wheat bread, 1 slice	1.4
Legumes, cooked	
Kidney beans, ½ cup	7.3
Lima beans, ½ cup	4.5
Vegetables, cooked	
Green peas, ½ cup	3.6
Corn, ½ cup	2.9
Potato, with skin, 1 medium	2.5
Broccoli, ½ cup	2.2
Lettuce, 1 cup	0.8
Fruits	
Apple, 1 medium	3.5
Orange, 1 medium	2.6
Banana, 1 medium	2.4
Dates, dried, 3	1.9
Peach, 1 medium	1.9

Adapted from Lanza E. Butrum R R: A critical review of food fiber analysis and data. J Am Diet Assoc 86:732, 1986.

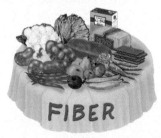

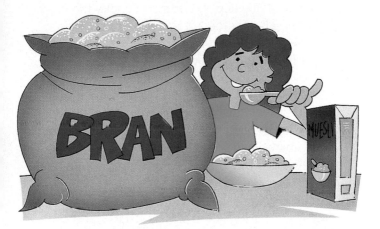

they should use a fiber-rich supplement such as wheat bran. Bran comes in many forms, some of which are very tasty. Natural wheat bran is very effective and versatile. A simple, pleasant, and inexpensive way of eating wheat bran is to mix it with hot or cold breakfast cereal. Bran also mixes well with thick soups, stewed apples, cooked rice, or yogurt, and quite well with orange juice. But don't spoil a nicely presented meal by sprinkling bran all over it!

Bran is available in health food stores and some supermarkets.

How much fiber is good?

Although the average fiber intake of Americans is only about 12 g a day, an intake of 20 to 35 g daily is advisable to promote regular, effortless bowel movements. This can be obtained from five to seven servings of vegetables and fruits, and generous amounts of whole-grain cereal or bread daily.

As with anything else, it is possible to take too much fiber. Some high-fiber foods upset certain people, making them feel bloated and uncomfortable or giving them diarrhea. If this is the case, they should use common sense and try a different food.

If you are one of those sensitive people, make sure you allow your gut time to recover fully before you try another fiber-rich food. Anyone who is increasing their intake of fiber should expect to pass more gas, but fortunately this unwanted side effect often diminishes after a few weeks.

Another way of getting into trouble with fiber is to increase your intake of it too quickly. If you want to change your diet, do it gradually so that your gut has time to get used to it. If you want to take wheat bran, start with a small dose, say one teaspoon a day, and increase it gradually over two to four weeks until you get the desired effect.

When to seek advice

If you have increased fiber intake substantially and still have problems, you should consult your doctor about alternatives. If wheat bran upsets you, try taking it in a different form such as bran-enriched bread or cereals (there are several brands) or even bran tablets.

If all types of bran upset you, then see your doctor.

Am I eating enough fiber?

People often ask how to know whether they are taking enough fiber. An intake of 20 to 35 g (just over or under an ounce) a day promotes regular, effortless bowel movements. You can modify your diet to include this much fiber by using the table or reading the fiber content printed on packages of cereal and other foods.

The appearance of your stools can also be a good indicator. If they are usually type 4 or close to it (refer to Bristol Stool Form Scale on page 17) you are probably getting enough.

KEY POINTS

■ Do not ignore a routine bowel urge, especially in the morning—this is what your bowels naturally prefer

■ Bowels are sensitive to stress and disruption of routine

■ Plenty of fiber in the diet
  —makes the stools bulkier and easier to pass
  —encourages the production of more disease-preventing acids in the colon

■ Fiber comes from plant cell walls and is available naturally in the diet from unprocessed plant food

What can go wrong?

Relief or frustration?

When everything goes right, bowel movements are one of the minor pleasures of life. As with a good scratch, they bring a a feeling of relief and satisfaction. In an ideal world, this brief but pleasant experience would

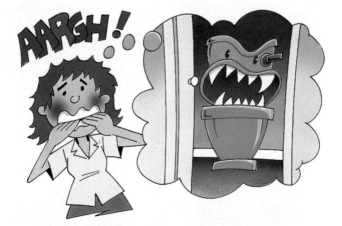

occur regularly, perhaps after getting up in the morning or after breakfast or another meal. The act of defecation would be predictable and effortless—quickly done and quickly forgotten. The reality is quite different for many people.

Straining

For many, getting started is an effort, nearly half the time people have to hold their breath and push or strain. Finishing is then unsatisfactory; often a feeling remains that the bowel had not emptied itself properly. In a survey of women who recorded their bowel habit for a month, every single one experienced this feeling of rectal dissatisfaction at some time in the month, and several women had it nearly every time they went.

The natural reaction to this feeling is to keep straining in the hope that something else will come out. But it doesn't. So there must be a lot of frustrated people behind the bathrom doors.

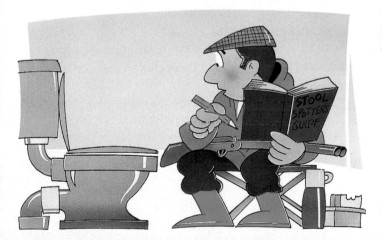

Another feeling that makes people strain is a feeling of needing to "go" but not being able to; when they try, they can't—there's nothing there.

Such false alarms are a common experience but, oddly, they have not been recognized as a symptom by enough doctors. Such experiences add to the widespread impression that defecation is an act that is unpredictable and uncomfortable—at best, a nuisance and, at worst, a nightmare.

Why are problems so common?
This is very odd. No other function of the body (except, perhaps, menstruation) regularly evokes such difficulty and such distress. We breathe unconsciously (except maybe after strenuous exercise), we eat and drink automatically or with pleasure, we usually urinate without thinking about it. Why should defecation be so different?

There are several reasons and it is important to understand them if one is to make sense of the irritable bowel syndrome (IBS) and other disorders.

Coming out of the closet
Defecation is the one human function that is often not discussed in public. When defecation is mentioned it is with a snigger, a giggle, a laugh, or a leer. All this makes it very difficult for someone who has a problem with defecation, or who just thinks they may have a problem, to mention it to anyone else. Fear of ridicule is a great conversation stopper.

Another problem with talking about defecation is that, for once, the English language is totally inadequate. Let us suppose someone decides to go to the doctor and tries to explain what is wrong. What

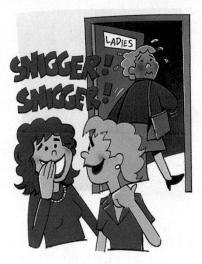

do they say? Usually, it is something rather vague like
"I can't go properly."

The doctor needs details

Let us suppose then that the doctor has figured out that
his/her patient has a problem with passing stools. How
does the interview go? Rather badly in many cases . . .

When patients say "I can't go properly" they could
mean at least five different things:

- I have to strain to start passing a stool

- I am not getting the urge to go as often as I think
  I should

- My stools are smaller than they should be

- I am getting false alarms, in other words,
  unproductive bowel urges

- When I have passed a stool, I feel as if there is
  something still inside the rectum.

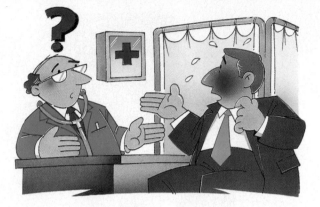

Why so much detail?

It is important for patients to get across to the doctor
what they really mean because the first two
symptoms—straining and inadequate urges—generally
mean the stool is abnormally small or hard. In other
words, there is constipation. This is actually described by
the third statement. The last two symptoms can be due
to constipation but are more often the result of an
irritable rectum (see irritable bowel syndrome, IBS,
page 82). A rectum can become irritable because it is
inflamed (proctitis) or because the patient has IBS.

So there are three main possibilities. Sorting them out
is a very practical problem because the exact symptom is
often a clue to the diagnosis. Treatment for constipation
won't help proctitis and it can even make IBS worse.

Problems with diagnosis

It would be best if all doctors were trained to sort out
these problems but, unfortunately, many are not.
Medical textbooks are largely silent on the subject of
stools and defecation, and medical students are taught

practically nothing about what is normal and what is abnormal. It is surprisingly uncommon for doctors, even specialists, to elicit such details from patients.

There are some bowel symptoms that have never been given a name and others whose definition varies in different dictionaries and textbooks. This unsatisfactory situation has arisen because very little scientific work has been done in the area of defecation and stools, so this part of medicine is underdeveloped.

What are the symptoms of bowel disorders?

When the bowel is diseased or malfunctioning, it usually draws attention to itself in one or more of the following ways:

- pain in the abdomen
- pain in the rectum or anus
- bloated feelings or actual swelling of the abdomen
- difficult passage of stools

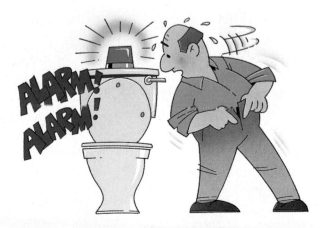

- hard stools
- less frequent passage of stools
- more frequent passage of stools
- loose or liquid stools
- feelings of incomplete emptying of the rectum
- urgency of need to pass stools
- passage of blood with the stool
- passage of mucus (slime) from the rectum
- appearance of a lump at the anus.

KEY POINTS

- Easy, regular passing of stools is a pleasure denied to us on at least some occasions in our lives

- Embarrassment about discussing bowel problems makes it difficult for the doctor to do something about them

- Problems can be caused by
  —constipation
  —inflamed rectum
  —irritable bowel syndrome (IBS)
  —rarer and serious diseases

Constipation

What is it?

Constipation is one of those words that everyone understands but is hard to define. It is often described as a symptom but, at best, it is a group of symptoms that vary from person to person. It is probably best defined as the state in which two things are objectively

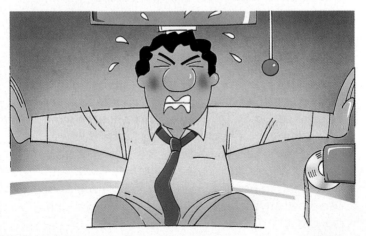

and measurably wrong: the output of stool is too low and the rate of passage of the colon's contents is too slow. Too little and too slow. Unfortunately, this definition is not useful in everyday life.

How do I know it's constipation?

Measuring stool output and passage time with any accuracy are just too difficult. Luckily, there is a third feature of constipation that is objective but is also easy to observe—the form or appearance of the stools. In constipation, the stool is lumpy —type 1 or type 2 on the Bristol Stool Form Scale (see page 17).

Apart from the form of the stools, the only reliable pointer to the state of constipation is infrequent defecation. Anyone who goes less than three times a week has slow transit. However, going more often is no guarantee that transit time is normal. It is possible to go every day, but every day be passing a stool that should have been passed three days before! There are even people who pass small, round lumps several times a day and think they have diarrhea. What they really have is constipation.

How common is it?

Surveys show that about 15% of North Americans have constipation, and it is at least twice as common in women as men. It is worse in pregnancy and just before a period, which are the times when the female sex hormone levels in the blood are at their highest. Severe, continuous constipation is almost unheard of in men, but affects at least one in 200 young women.

It seems to become more common as people age. Decreased physical activity, certain medications, and reduced intake are some of the reasons.

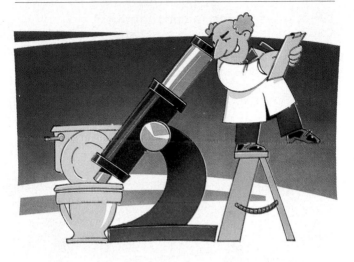

Problems of small, lumpy stools

A small stool does not stretch the rectum enough to generate a clear signal that you need to go; the urge to evacuate is weak. When the urge is weak, many people ignore it and postpone visiting the toilet.

Build up

This is bad news because an ignored urge goes away. What probably happens is that the ignored stool dries out and shrinks even more. Being smaller it needs to be reinforced by more stool before it is big enough to generate a signal again. Getting reinforcements takes time, so it is often several hours, sometimes a whole day, before another urge is felt. Ignoring the urge to pass stool or resisting it can definitely cause constipation.

Hard to shift

The smaller the stool is the more difficult it is to pass. It is as if the muscles cannot get hold of it, rather like a

What goes wrong in constipation?

Constipation is caused mainly by feces spending too long in the colon. During this extended period of time, the body continues to absorb water from the feces, making them hard, dry and difficult to propel and expel.

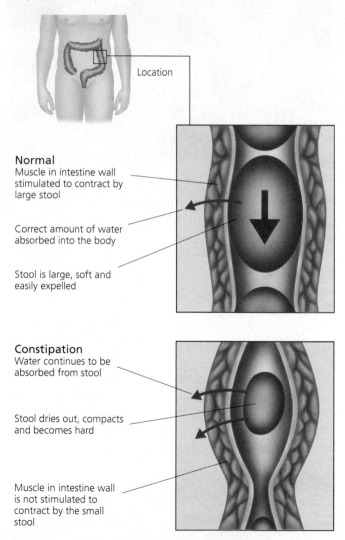

Location

Normal
Muscle in intestine wall stimulated to contract by large stool

Correct amount of water absorbed into the body

Stool is large, soft and easily expelled

Constipation
Water continues to be absorbed from stool

Stool dries out, compacts and becomes hard

Muscle in intestine wall is not stimulated to contract by the small stool dime that is too small for our fingers to hold. When a small stool expands by reinforcement over 24 hours it can turn into a hard, dry ball. Such a ball can be hard to pass. Moreover, straining to pass it can split the lining of the anal canal (fissure) and lead to pain and bleeding.

Straining and hemorrhoids
Straining—that is, holding the breath and pushing down—is often the only way to get rid of lumpy stools, but straining can be overdone. If you strain too hard or too long you can push out the soft cushions that seal the anal canal so that they protrude from the anus. This is what hemorrhoids (or piles) are (see page 93). Occasionally, even the lining of the rectum can be pushed out (rectal prolapse). So straining should be avoided or kept as brief as possible.

Rectal prolapse
A small rectal prolapse is particularly troublesome because, as it protrudes in the anal canal, it can make you feel as if a stool is still there. So you keep straining, which makes matters worse. This may be why some people with small stools never feel they have emptied their bowel completely.

Myths about constipation
Some long-held beliefs simply do not stand up under scientific scrutiny. The idea that constipation causes "autointoxication" by causing poisons to be absorbed into the bloodstream gained popularity about 100 years ago and still induces some people to obtain "high colonic" enemas from nonscientific practitioners, but this is merely a waste of time and money. There are

reasons to encourage a high fluid intake, but medical experiments have failed to show that colonic irrigation has any benefit for constipation or general well being.

How to cope with small or lumpy stools

Prevention is better than cure and there are several things you can do if you have difficulty with small and lumpy stools:

1 Always obey the urge to pass stool; in other words, if you feel the urge to go, go! Don't suppress it or delay going for more than a few minutes.

2 If possible, have a regular early morning routine so that, every day, what you do and when you do it is the same in the first hour after getting up.

3 Give yourself time to have a bowel movement in the morning before leaving home. If necessary, get up half an hour earlier.

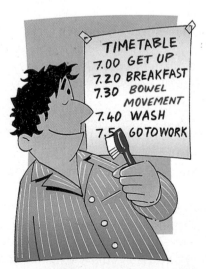

TIMETABLE
7.00 GET UP
7.20 BREAKFAST
7.30 BOWEL MOVEMENT
7.40 WASH
7.5 GO TO WORK

4 Eat breakfast. This is the best stimulus to a bowel movement.

5 Let your breakfast be substantial and rich in fiber. Some examples of such a breakfast are:

- a big bowlful of Shredded Wheat, wheat flakes, or bran flakes
- a bowl of All-Bran
- a bowl of granola with a tablespoonful of wheat bran mixed into it
- two slices of whole-wheat bread or toast, preferably made from a dense, chewy loaf (made from stone-ground flour).

Any of the above can be usefully supplemented with an apple or other fresh fruit (not just fruit juice) or some stewed dried fruit. Prunes are especially effective.

6 Make sure that the rest of your meals are rich in fiber (see page 46).

7 A tip about coping with difficulty in evacuation that so often results from the stool being small or hard: when sitting on the toilet, try placing your feet on a platform 4–8 inches high so that your thighs are nearer your chest. This makes the position nearer the squatting posture.

In some people small, lumpy stools are a reaction to stress or more accurately a sign of emotional tension. People who react like this are often dogged, determined types who do not readily show their emotions. It is as if, by holding onto their emotions, they hold onto their motions! Their gut reaction to stress is to slow down the passage of stool through the

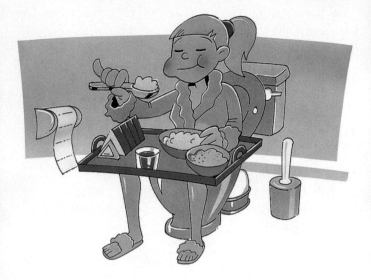

colon. If you react like this, you will improve only if you properly manage your tension or distress.

Laxatives

Anything that speeds up the passage of bowel contents and makes the stools softer or looser can be called a laxative or purgative.

Bulking agents

The most natural laxatives are the ones that work in the same way as dietary fiber—the so-called bulking agents. They are also the safest as they hardly ever cause watery diarrhea. There is little to choose between them except for taste and convenience. Several popular ones are available in handy packets,

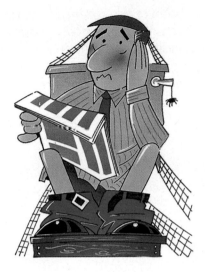

caplets, tablets, or wafers (Metamucil, Citrucel, or Fibercon). It is reasonable for people who think they are constipated to first increase their dietary fiber, and then try a bulking agent before consulting a doctor.

If you try a bulking agent, remember it works slowly. Take it for at least a week before deciding whether it works. If a small dose, say two packages a day, does not work, try three or four a day for a week before giving up. You may feel bloated for the first few weeks but this feeling should pass with time.

Stronger laxatives

A huge variety of stronger laxatives is available, many of which are based on traditional herbal remedies. However, don't be fooled into thinking that because a remedy is herbal in origin, and therefore "natural," it works like dietary fiber. On the contrary, many of these preparations, including some in herbal teas that are not clearly labeled as laxatives, work by stimulating the colon. Although it is unclear whether long-term use of such laxatives is dangerous, some of them stain the colon lining brown or gray. One thing is certain, and that is that dietary fiber and bulking agents are known to be safe.

As odd as it may seem, some constipated people actually feel more constipated when they increase dietary fiber or take a bulking agent; this is most common when the problem is long-term or severe. If this happens to you, it is alright to take senna or bisacodyl tablets from the pharmacy until you can see your doctor. You may need a physician's help.

Helping your doctor help you

If you go to see a doctor about constipation, keep a record of all your bowel movements for a week or two beforehand to show him/her. Recording the date and time of each bowel movement and the type of each stool, using the Bristol Stool Form Scale (see page 17), can give the doctor a clearer understanding of what you are experiencing. Make a note of how much you have to strain (hold your breath and push down). If it is longer than a minute or two, time it with your watch. Tell the doctor about any feelings of incomplete emptying and, if you are a woman, about variations in your bowel habit according to the time of the month. If you have recently taken any medications (including laxatives), take them along with you or, at least, details

Tips for avoiding constipation

If you have a tendency to be constipated you can help yourself in several ways:

- Maintain a high intake of dietary fiber, especially wheat fiber
- If possible, have a regular routine in the morning
- Eat breakfast
- Allow your bowels time to work in the morning
- Never ignore the feeling that you need to have a bowel movement. A suppressed urge can take many hours to return
- If your toilet seat is high, try putting your feet on a box or a pile of bricks or books
- If you're traveling, take some bran or bulking agent (Metamucil, Citrucel, or Fibercon)

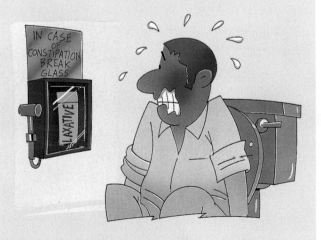

of their names and doses. Some drugs prescribed for high blood pressure, depression, and pain (narcotics or analgesics) as well as iron supplements can cause constipation.

Laxative-resistant constipation

In recent years, it has been recognized that some women (and, rarely, men) cannot defecate because they cannot relax the muscles in the floor of the pelvis that keep the anal canal closed or actually contract them when they should relax them. In short, they cannot "let go." And they may not be generating adequate force from their abdominal muscles to help expel stool.

It is almost as if they work against themselves to have bowel movements. Ordinary treatments do not help these people. Extra fiber just makes them feel bloated. Laxatives just cause pain or

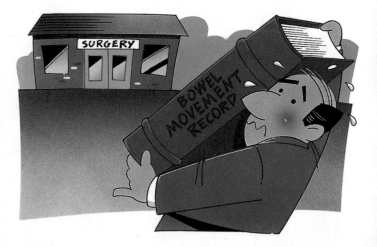

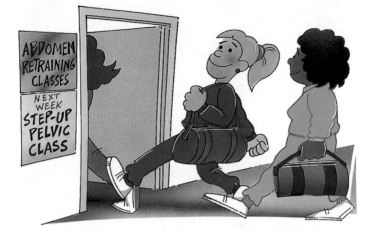

work only if taken in such big doses as to cause diarrhea.

There is a treatment that helps such people. It involves retraining their abdominal and pelvic muscles so that they cooperate instead of fighting against each other, utilizing a technique called biofeedback. Unfortunately, many doctors do not know about this therapy, and it is sometimes difficult to find someone, usually a physician or physical therapist, who can provide it. However, the situation should improve as the value of this treatment becomes accepted by more and more doctors.

Another reason why some women cannot push out a stool they know to be there is that, when they strain, the rectal wall bulges forward into the vagina and the stool gets jammed in the bulge. This can be cured by a surgical operation.

KEY POINTS

- You are constipated if you pass lumpy or hard stools, or have a bowel movement less than three times a week

- Avoiding constipation:
  —never ignore the urge to have a bowel movement
  —if possible, establish a morning routine
  —remember the fiber

- Laxatives: start with the bulking agents— mildest but slowest—before moving onto the stronger ones.

- See your doctor if you need strong laxatives regularly

- Go to your doctor if you develop constipation for no obvious reason, especially if you are over 40 (see page 100 for what the doctor is likely to do)

Diarrhea

What is it?

Diarrhea means passing liquid stools, that is, mushy or watery stools (type 6 or 7 on the Bristol Stool Form Scale, see page 17). It is not merely increased stool frequency, unless the stools are liquid as well.

Having to pass solid stools frequently is quite common and is a symptom of irritable bowel

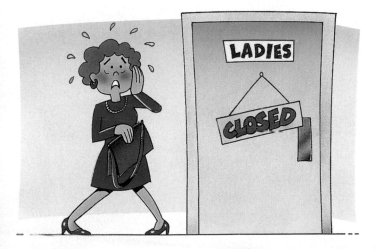

syndrome. There is no official name for it, but it could be called "pseudodiarrhea." The distinction is important because, in terms of cause and treatment, pseudodiarrhea and true diarrhea are quite different.

To the sufferer who never looks into the toilet bowl, they may seem exactly the same. To the doctor, the appearance of the stool is all-important so, if you plan to visit a doctor about what seems like diarrhea, make a note of what you see in the toilet before you go.

Liquid stools are liquid because they have traveled fast through the colon, whose job it is to absorb water and salts, or—much less commonly—because the colon is diseased. When liquid stools arrive in the rectum, you know about it at once, and in no uncertain terms. The urge to evacuate is so strong it can be painful. You have to drop everything and go to the toilet at once. Technically called "urgency of defecation," this symptom causes much distress, destroying social life and self-confidence.

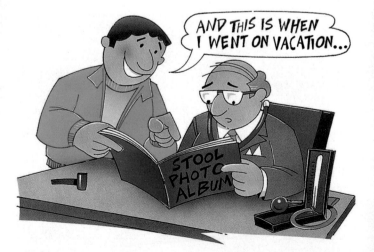

An even more distressing result of diarrhea is incontinence or soiling of the underclothes. It occurs because liquid seeps through the anus or, in the worst scenario, because the sufferer cannot get to the toilet in time—the rectal muscles have been too strong for the closing mechanisms of the anus. Incontinence is more common than people suppose. It is so embarrassing and disgusting to the sufferer that most do not mention it to their doctor unless asked directly, and many doctors do not ask.

How to cope with an attack of diarrhea

A single watery stool that spatters the pan is no cause for concern. Several such stools constitute an attack of diarrhea.

Luckily, most attacks settle by themselves. They settle more quickly if you lie down, keep warm, and avoid solid food for a few hours or a day or two. If it does not stop in three or four hours it is sensible to take an anti-diarrhea medication such as loperamide (Imodium

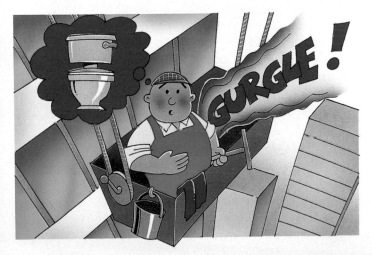

A-D), but the most important thing is to keep up your fluid intake so that you do not get dehydrated.

Water is absorbed best if it contains a little sugar and salt. Pharmacies sell rehydration powders containing balanced amounts of sugar and salts, and these come with full instructions. In an emergency you can drink lemonade or make your own rehydration solution (see Travelers' diarrhea).

If there is repeated vomiting as well as diarrhea, you should get medical help urgently. If diarrhea persists for more than a few days you should see a doctor.

You should seek medical advice without delay if:

- there is blood in the stool
- you are ill with fever
- the stool is black like tar.

Repeated diarrhea and how to cope with it

Diarrhea that keeps coming and going is most often due to irritable bowel syndrome, but other disorders can cause it, such as colitis and celiac sprue, a disease of the small intestine. You should see your doctor to be sure you don't have one of these less common disorders.

Healthy intestines sometimes rush their contents through. Why? There are many reasons for intestinal hurry but the most common is stress or anxiety. Many people get diarrhea before an exam, an interview, or any other challenging experience. It is part of the normal fight-or-flight response of a healthy body but in some people it occurs inappropriately often.

Intestinal hurry has many causes and the cure must depend on the cause. Eating the wrong foods and

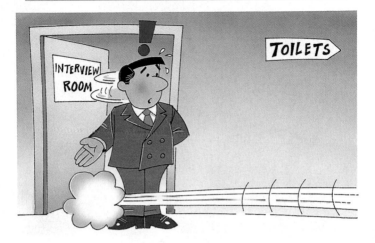

eating too much food can cause intestinal hurry. So can alcohol in some people, especially beer in large amounts. Many people have a certain food or drink that upsets them. If you know that eating a strong curry or drinking beer or milk leads to loose stools then,

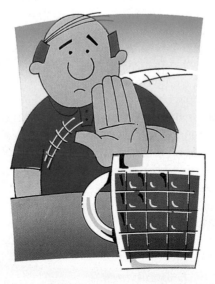

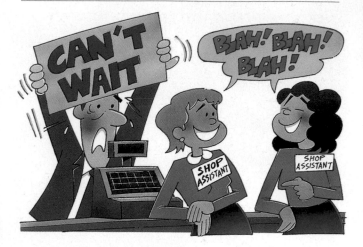

obviously, you should avoid them—unless you are happy to take the consequences!

If you have diarrhea in bouts, and food and drink don't seem to be responsible, then ask yourself if the bouts coincide with periods of stress in your life. If so, take action to reduce the stress or get teaching on how to handle stress better.

A short bout of diarrhea is not a serious threat to health. Persistent diarrhea is another matter and should trigger a visit to the doctor.

Some people believe in rice cakes and live yogurt. None of these has been tested scientifically but we are all different and, if something works for you and is safe, use it! Some people just need to eat less.

Should you still be prone to urgent, loose stools after doing all that you can think of, don't panic! To do so only makes things worse. To save embarrassment, plan your outings at times when you feel safest and consider taking a dose of loperamide (Imodium A-D) before leaving home.

KEY POINTS

- Diarrhea means passing liquid stools

- Most attacks settle by themselves

- For diarrhea that keeps coming and going, there are many possible causes, both psychological and physical

- Always consult a doctor if your diarrhea is persistent, bloody, or black (see page 100 for what the doctor is likely to do)

Bloating

Women especially

Up to 30% of people report bloating. Although some men have bloating, it is more likely to be a problem for women, either with or without other bowel symptoms. One survey revealed that 75% of women with IBS (see next section) had bloating. Typically, they say the abdomen is flat in the morning but becomes more distended as the day progresses. Some exclaim to the doctor, "I look like I am 6 months pregnant." Measurements have sometimes confirmed an increase in abdominal girth throughout the day—up to 5 inches (12 cm)! This often worsens around the time of menstrual periods.

What causes bloating?

There is a lot of confusion about this because, as with irritable bowel syndrome, there are multiple underlying causes that differ from person to person. Although x-rays may show increased intestinal gas, this is not clearly related to the feeling of bloating. A more consistent finding is that gas is moved through the bowel too slowly, just as delayed movement of bowel content causes constipation. People with deficient ability to digest lactose may have bloating if they drink milk—it usually takes more than 8 ounces (1 cup) to produce this reaction.

Researchers have found increased sensitivity to gas in the intestine of bloaters compared with non-bloaters, and also relaxation of bloaters' abdominal

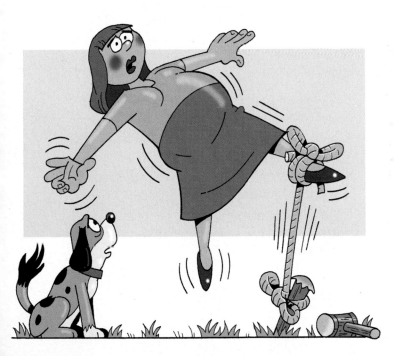

muscles, which results in abdominal protrusion. The cause or causes may differ from person to person, and tests in research laboratories would be needed to identify them.

Constipation and bloating

Constipation often increases the bloating sensation and, worse yet, the bran and bulking agents used to prevent constipation can worsen bloating. If this happens to you, consider asking your doctor for advice on managing the constipation.

What can be done?

It is unfortunate that for most people this common problem has no cure—many women would like to see the Nobel Prize awarded to the person who discovers one! Nevertheless, some simple, safe steps might help:

- Try reducing dietary fiber and gas-forming foods, such as beans and broccoli

- Reduce fructose (soft drinks) and avoid sorbitol (found in "sugarless candy")

- Try restricting milk but take a calcium supplement if you continue restriction

- Do not overeat; many bowel symptoms are worsened by eating too much at one time

- Take a walk after eating; mild physical activity increases gas movement through the bowel

KEY POINTS

■ Bloating is a very common symptom

■ Bloating is more frequent in women than men

■ There is no single cause of bloating; there are multiple underlying causes that vary from person to person

Irritable bowel syndrome (IBS)

What is it?

This is the name given by doctors to a group of chronic bowel symptoms—mainly abdominal pain or discomfort, altered bowel habit (diarrhea, constipation, or both), and bloating—that occur without any apparent disease of the intestines to explain them.

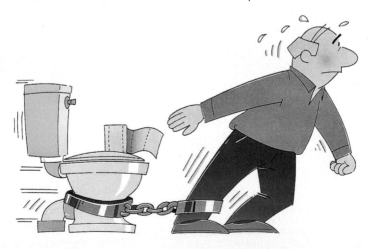

Short, self-limited spells of intestinal malfunction are common and part of normal life (see table on page 87). Surveys in many countries have revealed that about 10 to 20% of people have longer-lasting symptoms typical of IBS. It is often only a minor nuisance, but it can be bad enough to interfere with normal living.

What causes it?

This is not an easy question to answer because there are many causes. Usually, there seems to be more than one contributing factor. Some people have abnormally strong contractions of the intestines that cause a cramp like a leg muscle spasm. Excessive sensitivity in the intestines is another factor that has been proven experimentally when a balloon distended in the rectum of patients with IBS caused pain but the same amount of distension in people without bowel symptoms was painless. Sensitivity to certain foods—usually not an actual allergy like asthma—can sometimes worsen the problem. Depression or anxiety that might accompany problems with personal relationships or death of a loved one often worsen IBS. Some people have an episode of intestinal infection, such as travelers' diarrhea (see page 108), which leaves the intestines sensitive and IBS develops. The causes in one person often differ from those in someone else.

After signals from the intestine reach the brain, what the conscious mind perceives is influenced by the part of the brain that becomes activated in response to them. The signals—or even the anticipation of them before they occur—can be perceived as unpleasant feelings such as pain, bloating, or the urge to pass stool. But if they reach another part of the brain, the signals can be dampened so they do not seem as bothersome or are not perceived as unpleasant at all.

Focusing attention on part of the body makes it easier for signals from that part to reach the conscious mind, which can cause a vicious cycle. If you have a slight itch on your back and you focus your mind on it, it becomes a stronger itch. If you have a twinge somewhere and focus on it, it can turn into a pain. All sensations from the body can be amplified by this attention and, conversely, they can be reduced or even abolished by focusing on something else.

More women than men seek help from doctors for IBS. Although researchers are just beginning to find the answers to this puzzling fact, the reasons may have to do with different patterns of brain reactions to pain in women and men.

How can I be sure it is not serious?

Many people who go to a doctor with IBS are afraid there is something seriously wrong such as cancer, colitis, or ulcers. If you have IBS symptoms, you should consult a physician, especially if there is unintended weight loss, rectal bleeding, or frequent awakening at night with pain or diarrrhea, as these features suggest another explanation. However, some typical aspects of IBS are strong evidence that the problem is not due to serious disease.

1 The symptoms usually come and go over hours or days. For example, bloating or swelling of the abdomen gets worse as the day goes on but disappears overnight. In serious disease, the symptoms are persistent. There are a few exceptions such as the pain of gallbladder stones, but chronic diarrhea and constipation cannot be blamed on gallstones.

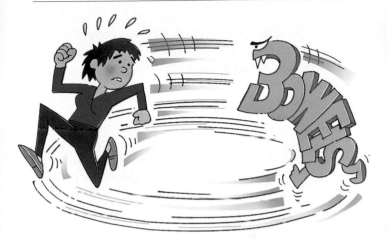

2 The symptoms of IBS vary from time to time. For
example, the pain is often felt in different places,
and the stools vary in appearance from day to day. In
serious disease, the symptoms tend to be less
variable.

3 The pain of IBS has features that indicate it comes
from the intestine. Typically, the pain eases after
bowel movements. Commonly, someone with IBS
has a change in bowel habit at a time when the
pains are occurring; typically, the stools become
softer or more frequent. Of course, there are
serious diseases that can cause intestinal pain and
a change of habit, but they are rare compared with
IBS and are usually obvious in some other way, for
example, by causing bleeding, weight loss, or
vomiting.

4 In IBS there are often symptoms of an irritable rectum;
these are unproductive bowel urges ("want to but

can't"), and feelings after defecation that there is still something inside the rectum. (With the latter feeling there is a natural tendency to keep straining but this should be resisted as it can make matters worse.) Serious disease rarely causes these symptoms and, when it does, it usually causes bleeding.

5 You may see slimy material (mucus) on the stool or even have occasions when you pass nothing but mucus. This is nothing to worry about unless it is copious or there is blood too. It is simply the reaction of an irritated rectum.

6 Some people with IBS notice they have to pass urine more often. This is a sign that the bladder has become more sensitive, like the intestine. In women, the genital organs may become more sensitive too, so that sexual intercourse is painful.

7 In some people with IBS, the stomach becomes more sensitive so that they feel excessively full after normal-size meals or after food or drink that never used to upset them.

8 A lot of people feel tired and listless during attacks of IBS and feel generally lousy. They sometimes also have headaches, backaches, or insomnia.

Visiting the doctor

So you can see that people with IBS have a lot to complain about. When it comes to visiting a doctor this multiplicity of complaints can be both good and bad. The good side is that the variety and characteristic nature of symptoms help the doctor conclude that the problem is a functional one instead of a life-threatening disease. The bad side is that some doctors find patients with all of these complaints hard to care for.

Common causes of short-lived diarrhea and/or constipation

Cause	Diarrhea	Constipation
Men and women		
Disturbed morning routine		✓
Emotional stress	✓	✓
Change in diet	✓	✓
Too much alcohol	✓	
Food intolerance	✓	
Travelers' diarrhea	✓	
Weight-loss diet		✓
Virus infections, gastroenteritis	✓	
Antibiotic treatment	✓	
Other medications	✓	✓
Women only		
Before and during periods	✓	✓
Pregnancy		✓

In trying to reassure the patient they may let drop an unhelpful remark like "there is nothing wrong with you." This is incorrect. There *is* something wrong but it is abnormal functioning of the intestines, not a disease in the conventional sense of an infection or tumor. Even though IBS is not life-threatening, it can impair many aspects of daily life. It is a condition that even specialists do not fully understand. But this does not mean that nothing can be done about it.

What can be done about IBS?

The most important thing for patients to do is find a doctor who shows interest in helping them with their symptoms. There is no substitute for an empathetic physician who can explain the symptoms and provide individualized advice on how to manage them. Treatment varies according to the severity and circumstances of each person's disorder. For many people with IBS, especially those who have recently developed it, this education, reassurance, and advice can help a lot. However, there is no permanent and complete cure for most people. Rather, they must learn to cope with their chronic, fluctuating symptoms. One reassuring thing is that once IBS has been confidently diagnosed, another cause for the symptoms is rarely found even after many years. A change in symptoms, however, calls for a return to your doctor.

Diet

Some people need to change their diet. If particular foods or drinks have triggered attacks or worsened the symptoms, they should be avoided or limited. Beans, cruciferous vegetables (such as broccoli and cauliflower), dairy, and wheat products may increase bloating and other symptoms. Fructose, which is often present in large amounts in soft drinks, and coffee can contribute to diarrhea. For constipation, it often helps to eat more fiber-rich foods (see page 46), unless these cause bloating. For many patients, excessively large or fatty meals are a problem rather than specifically what they eat. Above all, eat regular, sensible meals without rushing and avoid unnecessarily restrictive diets. There is so much variation among people concerning how the diet affects symptoms that no rules apply to everyone beyond these guidelines.

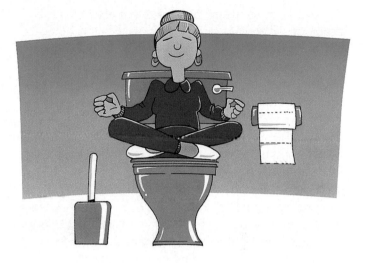

Medications

Medications are not the whole answer, but they can help specific symptoms. Over-the-counter loperamide (Imodium A-D) can reduce diarrhea and is especially useful when taken before meals or when leaving home to prevent the diarrhea that follows such activities. An older, prescription medication, diphenoxylate with atropine (Lomotil), works similarly. Bulking agents such as psyllium (Metamucil), methylcellulose (Citrucel), and calcium polycarbophil (Fibercon) may help constipation. Dicyclomine (Bentyl) or hyoscyamine (Levsin) are antispasmodic drugs that some people find useful for discomfort, but they can cause dry mouth and eyes and blurred vision. Antidepressant drugs in doses lower than needed for depression sometimes help pain and insomnia. Significant depression should be treated, as improvement in IBS often accompanies recovery from depression.

New drugs are being developed that affect the action of serotonin, a chemical "messenger" for sensations and bowel motility. However, many people are not helped by these drugs, and many physicians believe they should be limited to people with the most severe symptoms.

Psychotherapy

There is no human illness in which the mind-body interaction is more important than IBS. A variety of psychosocial therapies have shown promise, including individual or group psychotherapy, cognitive behavioral therapy, and hypnosis. Physicians select such treatment according to what they think will help and the patient's access to it, as determined by community availability and insurance coverage.

Lifestyle changes

Often people with IBS benefit from alterations in lifestyle that help them to relax and cope better with the stresses of life. Regular physical exercise helps a lot of people, as do yoga, tai chi, and meditation. For some people, the most important thing to do is to resolve problems of living, such as relationship or job issues, that make them tense, angry, or depressed.

Others simply need to take more time for relaxation and personal development. Each person has his or her own needs but may find it hard to objectively identify the problem areas. Here is where your physician or other professional can help. If you want a peaceful bowel, you need a peaceful mind!

KEY POINTS

- Irritable bowel syndrome (IBS) is a group of typical symptoms in the absence of abnormalities on diagnostic tests

- The mental attitude of the sufferer has a great influence on the severity of IBS

- Treatment can involve changes in lifestyle and diet; medication can also help, but the goal is coping, not curing

- Any single symptom of IBS can be caused by a serious disease so, if in doubt, check with your doctor

- See a doctor if you are losing weight or awakening at night because of pain or diarrhea

Bleeding from the anus

How common is it?

Bleeding from the anus after passing a stool is very common. At least 10% of people notice this, and of people who pay attention to their stools, particularly IBS sufferers, about 35% report seeing blood.

Where does it come from? In most people the blood comes from the anal canal and there are two common

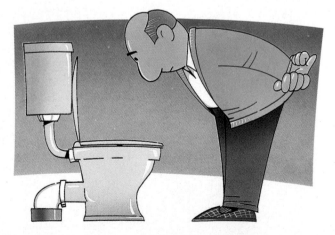

causes. Bleeding only once or a few times after passing an unusually large or hard stool is nearly always from a harmless small split or tear (fissure) in the lining of the anal canal. If there is no pain, the blood probably comes from a hemorrhoid (pile).

Hemorrhoids

A hemorrhoid is an anal cushion that has been pushed down the anal canal. It is a soft, fragile lump that is easily damaged when a stool passes over it. Often a person with a hemorrhoid does not know it is there, but some people can feel a lump just inside or outside the anus (see illustration on page 95). It may be uncomfortable but should not be painful. It may ooze a slimy material—mucus. This is a nuisance because it can soil the underwear and lead to itching around the anus.

The bleeding from an internal hemorrhoid can be quite alarming but it is rarely serious. It may splash or drip into the toilet water or just be seen as a streak on the stool or the toilet paper.

Hemorrhoids are caused by straining to pass a stool and so are most common in people who are constipated or who keep straining because the rectum is irritable, sending false signals that there is a stool inside.

Small hemorrhoids often go away when the constipation is cured or when straining stops. Bigger ones that bleed frequently need treatment. Usually a simple rubber band applied to the hemorrhoid makes it disappear but occasionally surgery is required.

When is bleeding serious?

In a small minority of people, bleeding is caused by a disease of the bowel higher up than the anus itself. The

most serious cause is cancer of the rectum or colon,
but bleeding can also come from innocent growths
(called polyps) and inflammation of the rectum
(proctitis) or the colon (colitis). If detected early enough,
cancer of the rectum or colon is curable. Polyps are
usually removed by colonoscopy, as otherwise a small
proportion of them enlarge over the years and become
cancerous. Proctitis and colitis require treatment with
medications administered orally or by enema or rectal
suppository.

The delicate structures around the anus

There are a lot of blood vessels in the walls of the anal canal
around the anus, and the lining is soft tissue with raised parts
called anal cushions or valves. These are delicate and can be
damaged by large or hard stools.

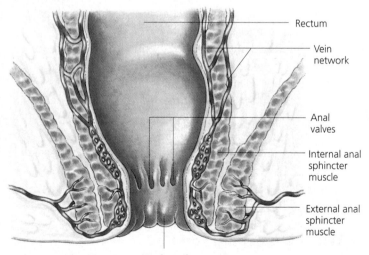

Rectum

Vein network

Anal valves

Internal anal sphincter muscle

External anal sphincter muscle

Anal canal

Bleeding from these causes may be less obvious than bleeding from the anus itself and may be seen only if you inspect the stool closely, or it may be invisible and only be detected by testing the stool (fecal occult blood test). If you see blood, you should see your doctor as soon as possible.

It is a sensible precaution for people over 50 to look at their stool occasionally, say once a month, to see if it shows blood. But don't be fooled by a piece of undigested tomato skin that looks like blood!

Types of hemorrhoid (piles)

The left-hand side of the picture shows normal anal cushions and the right-hand side shows hemorrhoids. They can be internal or external. Internal ones develop in the anal canal. External ones develop on the outer edge of the anus and may be visible.

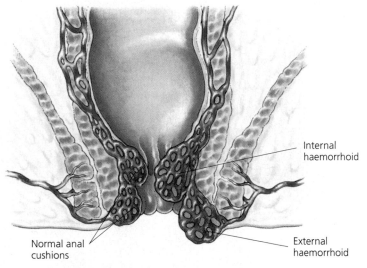

Internal haemorrhoid

External haemorrhoid

Normal anal cushions

The internal and external components of hemorrhoids.

KEY POINTS

■ Bleeding from the anus is common but only rarely indicates a serious problem. Tears in the anal canal or hemorrhoids are the usual explanation

■ But be on the safe side. See your doctor about bleeding as soon as you can

■ Regularly check for blood in the stool if you are over 50

Diverticulosis

What is it?

A diverticulum is a small pouch protruding through the wall of the colon. Most are about ¼ to ½ inch (5 to 10 mm) in diameter. If you have one, you nearly always have more, so you have diverticulosis. It increases as we grow older, and by age 80 about two-thirds of Americans will have diverticulosis.

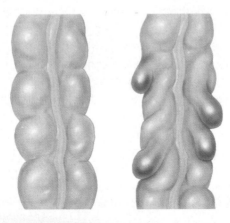

Why do we get it?

In the 1960s, researchers found that African villagers rarely had diverticulosis. What distinguishes them from city-dwellers, especially those in the industrialized countries, is their unrefined, high-fiber diet, which produces voluminous, bulky stools. The theory has developed that processed, low-fiber diets cause the muscles in the wall of the colon to contract vigorously to move fiber-deficient, small stools along and that this force causes the diverticula to bulge where the colon is weakest. This theory is difficult to prove, but it is supported by the finding of increased colonic motility (contractions) in people with diverticulosis.

How is it found?

Most people don't know they have it. Diverticulosis is usually discovered by a sigmoidoscopy, colonoscopy, or barium enema performed because of unrelated symptoms or as a colorectal cancer screening procedure. Many people with IBS have diverticulosis, but their symptoms are no different from those of people who have no diverticulosis. So for the most part, they are uncomplicated (do not cause illness).

Complications

A minority of people develop either diverticulitis or acute (sudden) bleeding from a diverticulum. Diverticulitis occurs when a diverticulum bursts and bacteria leak out around the colon, typically causing severe pain and fever. This should be treated with antibiotics, and occasionally an abscess (collection of pus) or other complication develops that requires drainage with a tube or surgery.

A diverticulum bleeds if an artery pokes through its

thin wall. This results in passage of lots of blood from the anus, which is obviously serious. After hospitalization, a blood transfusion is often needed, and colonoscopy or other tests are used to find where in the colon the bleeding diverticulum is located. Fortunately, the bleeding stops by itself in most cases. But a colectomy (surgical removal of part of the colon) is sometimes needed.

What should I do about it?

Diverticula do not go away, which is of little concern as most of them never cause problems. Whether a high-fiber diet prevents the development of more diverticula is unknown, but is advisable to prevent constipation and improve health in other ways. Also, it is unclear whether particulate food, such as nuts, seeds, and popcorn, get stuck in diverticula and cause diverticulitis—at least this sequence of events has not been proven. Many people are probably avoiding these foods unnecessarily, but if eating them clearly brings on symptoms, it makes sense to restrict them.

KEY POINTS

- The frequency of diverticulosis increases as we get older

- A high fiber diet is thought to reduce the likelihood of developing diverticulum

- Diverticulitis occurs when a diverticulum bursts and bacteria leak out around the colon

Physician evaluation and special tests

What will the doctor do?

Some people put off going to see a doctor with a bowel complaint for fear of what may be done to them. Actually it will not be as bad as they think. An internal examination may be undignified and uncomfortable but it should not be intolerably painful.

History taking

First the doctor will ask you to describe your bowel symptoms and any others and question you, if necessary, to fill in the details. "Taking the history" is a long tradition in medicine. Despite all the modern technological advances in diagnosis, the information you give the doctor is still the most important part of your medical evaluation. So try to explain what is wrong carefully—bring notes if that will help. Bring all of the medications, vitamins, and anything else you take, as this will show more accurately and quickly what you take than what you could tell the doctor from memory. If you have had other doctor visits or tests for the current problem and this doctor will not have records of them, it is very helpful to bring copies of the reports. This can help the doctor determine what you need and prevent unnecessary duplication of tests.

Physical examination

The doctor's examination will include examining the abdomen with you lying on your back; he or she will gently probe it, at first lightly, then quite deeply, searching the entire abdomen for any lumps or tender spots. The doctor will ask you to turn onto your left side with your knees drawn up for a rectal examination. After inspecting outside of the anus, he or she will feel inside it with a gloved finger lubricated with jelly. The doctor feels for growths in the anus and rectum and, in men, makes an important check for prostate abnormalities.

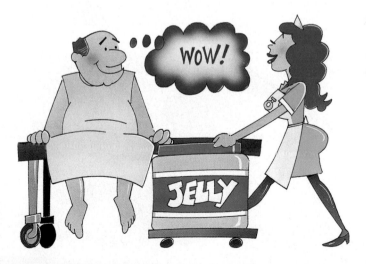

You can make the examination more comfortable and easier for the doctor by relaxing the muscles round the rectum. It helps if you breathe slowly and deeply with your mouth open. The examination is over soon.

After this examination and any laboratory tests that may be needed for specimens of your blood, urine, or stool, such as a fecal occult blood test (see the Glossary), the doctor may advise you to have one or more special internal examinations.

Anoscopy

The doctor may want to examine the anal canal and lower rectum with a four-inch long metal tube. If you relax your anus again, the tube will slide in just as easily as the examiner's finger because it is well lubricated and its end is rounded by a removable plug.

When the plug is pulled out a bright light shows the examiner if there are any hemorrhoids or other problems in the anal canal. These become obvious as the instrument is slowly pulled out. The tube may feel

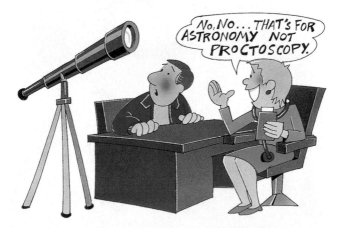

cold and strange but it should not hurt. If it does, say so at once as this might indicate you have a fissure and the examiner will stop.

Sigmoidoscopy

Another common examination is sigmoidoscopy. Most sigmoidoscopies are performed with a flexible endoscope (flexible sigmoidoscopy), through which a doctor or specially trained physician's assistant or nurse looks directly, or that transmits the image to a video screen. It permits a direct inspection of the lining of the rectum, sigmoid, and variable portions of the descending colon. This is a common colorectal cancer screening procedure.

You need to clear the lower bowel with enemas or laxatives before the procedure. Sigmoidoscopy usually takes only two or three minutes but it is very valuable. During the exam, you lie on your left side. The examiner must inject some air into the bowel. You may feel a sensation of needing to pass gas or stool when this is done.

While performing a sigmoidoscopy, the doctor may decide to take one or more small samples of tissue (biopsies) from the lining for examination under the microscope. This is done with an instrument passed down the tube. Most people feel nothing or only a minor sensation when biopsies are taken. Serious complications from flexible sigmoidoscopy are rare.

Colonoscopy

A colonoscopy is basically an extension of sigmoidoscopy, for which a longer endoscope is used that provides examination of the entire large intestine and even the lower small bowel (ileum). Thorough

Investigating the colon

Many abnormalities of the rectum and sigmoid colon can be seen by your doctor through a sigmoidoscope. This is a routine procedure that may cause slight discomfort, but it is unlikely to be painful.

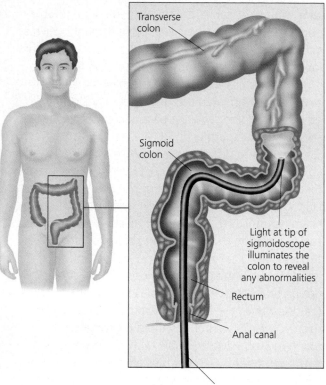

Transverse colon

Sigmoid colon

Light at tip of sigmoidoscope illuminates the colon to reveal any abnormalities

Rectum

Anal canal

Sigmoidoscope allows the doctor to see inside the rectum and sigmoid colon

colon preparation is required. Besides allowing biopsies, small growths (polyps) can be removed with electrocautery applied through a wire loop. Intravenous medication is usually given, which requires close monitoring of your pulse, blood pressure, and blood oxygen level. Discomfort is usually minor, but more severe pain sometimes occurs. The time required varies, but it averages about 20 minutes, and it can be prolonged by polyp removal or if your colon is more tortuous and difficult to traverse than usual.

Due to its ability to examine the entire large bowel, some physicians prefer it for colorectal cancer screening, especially if your risk is increased because one or more of your family members have had colorectal cancer. There is a small risk of bleeding after polyp removal or, worse and less often, perforation of the colon (often requiring emergency surgery). Doctors consider your age, general health, specific symptoms, and history of family illness before deciding whether you should undergo colonoscopy.

Barium enema X-ray

The other common test for bowel problems is an X-ray examination called a barium enema. This, too, requires clean-out preparation to eliminate stool that might confuse the result. You lie on your side on the X-ray table, and a lubricated tube is placed in your rectum. The radiologist pours a liquid suspension of barium sulfate through the tube and injects some air along with it. You will be asked to change your position several times so that the barium coats the entire colon lining. The barium shows up on X-ray films, permitting the detection of polyps or other abnormalities. Serious side effects are very rare.

Barium enema X-ray

Barium is administered through a tube into the patient's empty rectum. Barium is opaque to X-rays so it shows up on film, revealing any diseases or abnormalities of the large intestine.

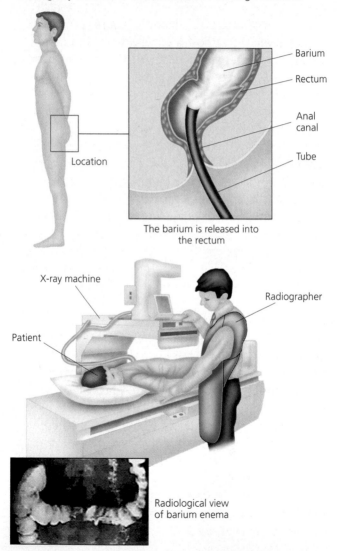

Location

Barium

Rectum

Anal canal

Tube

The barium is released into the rectum

X-ray machine

Radiographer

Patient

Radiological view of barium enema

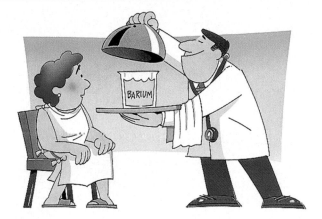

During this procedure, several X-ray films are taken. Finally the air and some barium are drained out and you are shown to the bathroom so you can pass some of the remaining barium. The rest of it passes over the next few days.

KEY POINTS

■ Your doctor will examine you both outside and inside. The inside examination should cause only minor discomfort.

■ Additional testing may include sigmoidoscopy, colonoscopy, or barium enema.

Travelers' problems

Travel changes bowel habit
A change in bowel function often occurs with travel.
Constipation is common with any type of travel, but
travelers to developing countries are more likely to
develop diarrhea, and it can be more disabling.

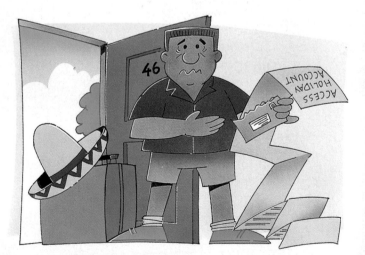

Constipation

There has never been a thorough investigation of this phenomenon, but many people have less frequent stools that are difficult to pass when they are away from home. There are several reasons why this may happen.

1 The travel schedule may interfere with prompt responses to bowel movement urges.

2 During long-distance travel with crossing of time zones, there is disruption of the internal or biological clock that controls human body rhythms.

3 There is a change of diet which, for many people, means a reduction in their intake of dietary fiber.

Some of this is inevitable. But there are steps you can take to prevent constipation when you are traveling.

1 When flying, choose an aisle seat on the plane that is easy to leave for the toilet.

2 Avoid sitting still for long periods; if you are driving, stop the car, and take a walk every hour or so.

3 Bring your own high-fiber food such as bread and cereal. More compactly, you can take packages of a bulking laxative (see page 64). Start to take it a day or two before you leave home.

4 When you have an urge to empty the bowels, make sure you respond to it as soon as possible.

Diarrhea

The risk of travelers' diarrhea depends on where you travel. Visits within the U.S. or to Canada, northern Europe, Australia, and New Zealand carry less than a

10% risk. The risk is 10 to 20% if you visit a Caribbean island, South Africa, and the Mediterranean, and it increases to above 30% (as high as 60%) in Mexico, South and Central America, and most of Asia and Africa.

Diarrhea with abdominal cramping and sometimes with vomiting can destroy at least part of a vacation or interfere with a business trip. The usual cause is water or food contamination with harmful bacteria or viruses; parasites are less common except in certain locales. Symptoms usually last 1 to 5 days. For mild diarrhea, any safe liquid (e.g., soft drinks without ice or broth) is recommended, and saltine crackers can provide salt. Severe diarrhea is more likely to cause dehydration, which is best prevented with oral rehydration powder purchased from a pharmacy on the trip or brought from home. It should be mixed with water that is known to be clean, according to the directions with the powder packets. Or you can make a substitute solution yourself with the following recipe:

4¼ cups (1 liter) water
½ teaspoon salt
½ teaspoon baking soda
4 tablespoons sugar

Antidiarrhea drugs are generally not recommended, as they do not kill bacteria and can give you the false sense of improvement by reducing stool frequency while fluid accumulates in your intestine, leading to dehydration. If you have more than 4 stools daily, fever, or blood or pus in your stools, it is likely an antibiotic would speed your recovery. Ciprofloxacin (Cipro) is often recommended and is worth taking on trips, as the sooner you start taking it, the quicker you will recover. However, bacteria are developing resistance to antibiotics in a race against the scientists who try to develop new antibiotics that can kill the bacteria. So the best antibiotic now might not be the ideal choice in the future—and where you plan to travel is also important. So you should get advice from a physician about what you should take. Visit a doctor if, despite treatment, you have symptoms for more than 10 days

The best approach is prevention, and there are a number of steps you can take to decrease the risk.

1 Drink only bottled water or nonalcoholic beverages, preferably from their original containers with a straw (glasses, cups, and the outside of bottles can be contaminated).

2 Boil water for 3 minutes or add 2 drops of household bleach or 5 drops of tincture of iodine to 4¼ cups (1 liter) water and wait 30 minutes (the water won't taste great, however!).

3 Avoid ice and mixed drinks (alcohol does not make the water safe).

4 Avoid milk unless you know it has been pasteurized.

5 Food should be thoroughly cooked.

6 Watch out for salads or buffet meals, as the food might have been inadequately washed, or prepared so long ago that bacteria have grown in it. Fruit you peel yourself should be safe.

7 Beware of uncooked sauces served separately from the food.

8 Remember that the food served on your departing flight comes from the place you are leaving and could be contaminated.

KEY POINTS

- Travel often causes constipation but simple precautions can prevent it

- Travelers' diarrhea is the result of contaminated food or drink

- In high risk areas, it is wise to take an antibiotic in case you need it

- Vigilance is required to prevent travelers' diarrhea

Glossary

Absorption: after digestion, the passage of water, minerals, and food components through the wall of the intestine into the bloodstream.

Anus: the lower opening of the gastrointestinal tract.

Barium enema: an X-ray procedure during which a thick, white liquid (a suspension of barium sulfate) is

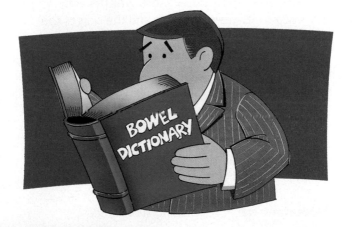

introduced into the colon via a tube in the anus. It is used to look for colitis, polyps, etc.

Biofeedback: a technique for training the body that is enhanced with "feedback" of the desired result, such as training of the pelvic floor while muscle activity is measured.

Bran: the outer coating of a cereal grain, usually wheat (after the husk has been removed). Bran is an exceptionally rich source of dietary fiber.

Colectomy: surgical removal of the colon.

Colitis: inflammation of the colon. The cause can be unknown or an infection.

Colonoscopy: examination of the colon by a flexible endoscope (colonoscope) which is introduced via the anus.

Colostomy: surgical procedure in which an opening is constructed between the colon and the skin of the abdomen.

Constipation: difficulty in passing stools and/or having lumpy stools.

Crohn's disease: a particular type of inflammation of the gastrointestinal tract, usually the lower small intestine and/or large intestine, that is chronic (long-lasting) and of unknown cause.

Defecation: the act of passing stools (feces).

Diarrhea: the passage of unusually loose (unformed) stools. It is often associated with increased frequency of defecation.

Digestion: breakdown of protein, carbohydrate, and fat by enzymes in the stomach and small intestine so the food can be absorbed.

Diverticulitis: infection around a burst colon diverticulum.

Diverticulosis: plural of "diverticulum."

Diverticulum: small pouch protruding from the wall of the colon.

Endoscopy: looking inside the body through an instrument, such as a colonoscope.

Enteric nervous system: a network of nerves in the intestinal wall that controls the function of the intestine.

Fecal occult blood test: a test performed on a small specimen of stool to determine if it contains invisible blood.

Fiber: the indigestible parts of plant foods, consisting mainly of cell walls that increase the bulk of stools.

Fissure, anal fissure: a split in the lining of the anal canal that usually cause pain and minor bleeding.

Flatulence: anal passage of gas ("fart").

Flatus: gas passed from the anus.

Functional gastrointestinal disorders: disorders characterized by symptoms induced by abnormal gastrointestinal function in the absence of structural (infections, tumor, ulcer, etc) or metabolic (diabetes, vitamin deficiency, etc) abnormalities; irritable bowel syndrome is the prototype.

Gastroenteritis: inflammation of the gastrointestinal tract.

Gastrointestinal tract: organs from the mouth to the anus through which food enters, is digested and absorbed, and the waste (stool) exits.

Gastroenterologist: specialist in diseases of the gastrointestinal tract.

Hemorrhoids (piles): soft swellings that start in the anal canal and may protrude from the anus and bleed.

Ileostomy: a surgical procedure in which an opening is constructed between the end of the small intestine (ileum) and the skin of the abdomen.

Incontinence: involuntary escape of stool from the anus (or of urine from the bladder).

Irritable bowel syndrome (IBS): a collection of symptoms that is caused by the bowel, especially the colon, being irritable; also called "spastic colon" and "spastic colitis."

Laxative: a product that helps to make passing stools easier and the stool softer.

Lumen: the space inside the bowel.

Mucosa: the lining of the bowel.

Organic gastrointestinal disorders: disorders caused by structural (infections, tumor, ulcer, etc) or metabolic (diabetes, vitamin deficiency, etc) abnormalities.

Peristalsis: a coordinated movement of gastrointestinal muscle activity that moves the bowel contents downward.

Polyp: a small growth, often on a stalk, arising from the lining of the intestine; usually benign unless large.

Probiotics: ingested bacteria that benefit health.

Proctitis: inflammation of the rectum.

Rectum: the last few inches of the bowel, above the anal canal.

Sigmoid: the last part of the colon, above the rectum.

Sigmoidoscopy: examination of the rectum and sigmoid by an optical or computerized instrument called a sigmoidoscope, which is introduced via the anus.

Travelers' diarrhea: sudden, short-lived attack of diarrhea caused by bacteria or viruses in contaminated food or beverages taken during travel, especially to developing countries.

Useful addresses

Where can I learn more?

We have included the following organizations because, on preliminary investigation, they may be of use to the reader. However, we do not have first-hand experience of each organization and so cannot guarantee the organization's integrity. The reader must therefore exercise his or her own discretion and judgment when making further inquiries.

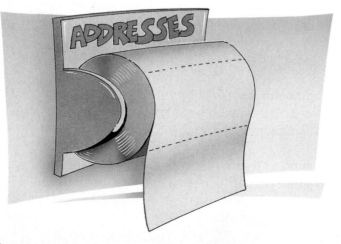

American College of Gastroenterology (www.acg.gi.org)
Professional organization with web site that includes Patient Information.

American Gastroenterological Association (www.gastro.org)
Professional organization with web site that includes Patient Center.

Centers for Disease Control and Prevention (www.cdc.gov/travel/)
Details health risks and gives illness prevention and treatment advice for travel throughout the world.

Center for Science in the Public Interest (www.cspinet.org)
Independent non-profit consumer health group that provides practical, scientific information on nutrition. Publication available by subscription.

International Foundation for Functional Gastrointestinal Disorders (www.iffgd.org)
Comprehensive source of information on various aspects of gastrointestinal function and functional disorders, including irritable bowel syndrome. Quarterly member publication and reprinted articles on many topics available.

MedlinePlus (www.medlineplus.gov)
U.S. National Institutes of Health and National Library of Medicine
Extensive information source, including recent medical research news and links to PubMed (medical article indexing and retrieval).

U.S. National Institutes of Health (www.health.nih.gov)
Extensive information on health, illnesses, and their diagnosis and treatment. Several publications by subscription.

Searching the internet as a source of further information

After reading this book, you may feel that you would like further information on the subject. The internet is, of course, an excellent place to look and many websites contain useful information about medical conditions, related charities, and support groups.

It should always be remembered, however, that the internet is unregulated and anyone is free to set up a website and add information to it. Many websites offer impartial advice and information that has been compiled and checked by qualified medical professionals. Some, on the other hand, are run by commercial organizations with the purpose of promoting their own products. Others still are run by pressure groups, some of which will provide carefully assessed and accurate information whereas others may be suggesting medications or treatments that are not supported by the medical and scientific community.

Unless you know the address of the website you want to visit—for example,www.webmd.com—you may find the following guidelines useful when searching the internet for information.

Search engines and other searchable sites

Google (www.google.com) is the most popular search engine used in the United States, followed by Yahoo! (www.yahoo.com) and MSN (www.msn.com). Also popular are the search engines provided by Internet Service Providers such as AOL (www.aol.com).

In addition to the search engines that index the whole of the web, there are also medical sites with search facilities, which act almost like mini-search engines, covering only medical topics or even a particular area of medicine. Again, it is wise to look at who is responsible for compiling the information offered to ensure that it is impartial and medically accurate.

Search phrases

Be specific when entering a search phrase. Searching for information on "cancer" will return results for many different types of cancer as well as on cancer in general. You may even find sites offering astrological information! More useful results will be returned by using search phrases such as "lung cancer" and "treatments for lung cancer." Both Google and Yahoo offer an advanced search option that includes the ability to search for the exact phrase; enclosing the search phrase in quotes, that is, "treatments for lung cancer," will have the same effect. Limiting a search to an exact phrase reduces the number of results returned but it is best to refine a search to an exact match only if you are not getting useful results with a normal search.

Always remember the internet is international and unregulated. It holds a wealth of valuable information but individual sites may be biased, out-of-date, or just plain wrong. Family Doctor Publications accepts no responsibility for the content of links published in this series.

Index

Your pages

We have included the following pages because they may help you manage your illness or condition and its treatment.

Before an appointment with a health professional, it can be useful to write down a short list of questions of things that you do not understand, so that you can make sure that you do not forget anything.

Some of the sections may not be relevant to your circumstances.

Health-care contact details

Name:

Job title:

Place of work:

Tel:

Name:

Job title:

Place of work:

Tel:

Name:

Job title:

Place of work:

Tel:

Name:

Job title:

Place of work:

Tel:

Significant past health events—illnesses/operations/investigations/treatments

Event	Month	Year	Age (at time)

Appointments for health care

Name:

Place:

Date:

Time:

Tel:

Name:

Place:

Date:

Time:

Tel:

Name:

Place:

Date:

Time:

Tel:

Name:

Place:

Date:

Time:

Tel:

Appointments for health care

Name:

Place:

Date:

Time:

Tel:

Name:

Place:

Date:

Time:

Tel:

Name:

Place:

Date:

Time:

Tel:

Name:

Place:

Date:

Time:

Tel:

Current medication(s) prescribed by your doctor

Medicine name:

Purpose:

Frequency & dose:

Start date:

End date:

Medicine name:

Purpose:

Frequency & dose:

Start date:

End date:

Medicine name:

Purpose:

Frequency & dose:

Start date:

End date:

Medicine name:

Purpose:

Frequency & dose:

Start date:

End date:

Other medicines/supplements you are taking, not prescribed by your doctor

Medicine/treatment:

Purpose:

Frequency & dose:

Start date:

End date:

Medicine/treatment:

Purpose:

Frequency & dose:

Start date:

End date:

Medicine/treatment:

Purpose:

Frequency & dose:

Start date:

End date:

Medicine/treatment:

Purpose:

Frequency & dose:

Start date:

End date:

Questions to ask at appointments
(Note: do bear in mind that doctors work under great time
pressure, so long lists may not be helpful for either of you)

Questions to ask at appointments
(Note: do bear in mind that doctors work under great time
pressure, so long lists may not be helpful for either of you)

Notes

Notes

Notes